COPING WITH INCO[N...]

DR JOAN GOMEZ is Honorary Consulting Psychiatrist to the Chelsea and Westminster Hospital. She was trained at King's College, London, and Westminster Hospital, qualifying MB, BS, and obtained her DPM in 1973 and MRCPsych in 1974. She was elected a Fellow of the Royal College of Psychiatrists in 1982, and obtained the Diploma in the History of Medicine in 1996 and the Diploma of the Philosophy of Medicine in 1998. She is a Fellow of the Society of Apothecaries and also of the Royal Society of Medicine. She has been engaged in clinical work and research on the interface between psychiatry and physical medicine. Dr Gomez is the author of several books published by Sheldon Press: *Coping with Thyroid Problems* (1994), *How to Cope with Bulimia* (1995), *Living with Diabetes* (1995), *How to Cope with Anaemia* (1998), *Coping with Gallstones* (2000), *Living with Crohn's Disease* (2000) and *Living with Osteoporosis* (2001). Her husband was a general practitioner and they have ten children.

Overcoming Common Problems Series

For a full list of titles please contact
Sheldon Press, Marylebone Road, London NW1 4DU

The Assertiveness Workbook
A plan for busy women
JOANNA GUTMANN

Birth Over Thirty Five
SHEILA KITZINGER

Body Language
How to read others' thoughts by their gestures
ALLAN PEASE

Body Language in Relationships
DAVID COHEN

Cancer – A Family Affair
NEVILLE SHONE

Coping Successfully with Hayfever
DR ROBERT YOUNGSON

Coping Successfully with Migraine
SUE DYSON

Coping Successfully with Pain
NEVILLE SHONE

Coping Successfully with Your Irritable Bowel
ROSEMARY NICOL

Coping with Anxiety and Depression
SHIRLEY TRICKETT

Coping with Breast Cancer
DR EADIE HEYDERMAN

Coping with Bronchitis and Emphysema
DR TOM SMITH

Coping with Chronic Fatigue
TRUDIE CHALDER

Coping with Depression and Elation
DR PATRICK McKEON

Curing Arthritis Diet Book
MARGARET HILLS

Curing Arthritis – The Drug-Free Way
MARGARET HILLS

Depression
DR PAUL HAUCK

Divorce and Separation
Every woman's guide to a new life
ANGELA WILLANS

Everything Parents Should Know About Drugs
SARAH LAWSON

Good Stress Guide, The
MARY HARTLEY

Heart Attacks – Prevent and Survive
DR TOM SMITH

Helping Children Cope with Grief
ROSEMARY WELLS

How to Improve Your Confidence
DR KENNETH HAMBLY

How to Interview and Be Interviewed
MICHELE BROWN AND GYLES BRANDRETH

How to Keep Your Cholesterol in Check
DR ROBERT POVEY

How to Pass Your Driving Test
DONALD RIDLAND

How to Start a Conversation and Make Friends
DON GABOR

How to Write a Successful CV
JOANNA GUTMANN

Hysterectomy
SUZIE HAYMAN

The Irritable Bowel Diet Book
ROSEMARY NICOL

Overcoming Guilt
DR WINDY DRYDEN

The Parkinson's Disease Handbook
DR RICHARD GODWIN-AUSTEN

Talking About Anorexia
How to cope with life without starving
MAROUSHKA MONRO

Think Your Way to Happiness
DR WINDY DRYDEN AND JACK GORDON

Overcoming Common Problems

Coping with Incontinence

Dr Joan Gomez

sheldon **PRESS**

First published in Great Britain in 2003 by
Sheldon Press
1 Marylebone Road
London NW1 4DU

Copyright © Joan Gomez 2003

All rights reserved. No part of this book may be reproduced
or transmitted in any form or by any means, electronic or
mechanical, including photocopying, recording, or by any
information storage and retrieval system, without permission
in writing from the publisher.

British Library Cataloguing-in-Publication Data

A catalogue record for this book is available from the British Library

ISBN 0–85969–900–5

1 3 5 7 9 10 8 6 4 2

Typeset by Deltatype Limited, Birkenhead, Merseyside
Printed in Great Britain by Biddles Ltd
www.biddles.co.uk

Contents

Introduction	vii
1 The waterworks – what they consist of and how they work	1
2 The big problem	6
3 The middle years	13
4 The male angle	20
5 Juniors	28
6 Adolescents	34
7 Seniors	38
8 Special problems – prolapse, fistula and fibroids	45
9 Pregnancy and childbirth	52
10 Checking out what's wrong	56
11 Coping – aids and appliances	63
12 Coping – medicines	68
13 Coping – surgical operations	77
14 Training your bladder – exercises	81
15 Faecal incontinence	88
16 Thoughts and feelings – the psychological aspect	92
17 Cystitis	97
18 Problems with passing water	105
19 Lifestyle	110
20 Outline of a day	122
21 Nourishment and repair	127
Further reading	141
Useful addresses	142
Index	147

Introduction

Incontinence is nothing new. It is mentioned by the Egyptians in the Ebers papyrus in around 1500 BC, and the ancient Greeks had several cures. One of the earliest prescriptions – 1550 BC – recommends a mixture based on cypress beans and juniper berries. An infusion of white chrysanthemums in lukewarm water, a powder made from burnt cocks' testicles, or attaching a frog to the patient's belt were other ploys.

In 1556, the London physician Thomas Phaer wrote a chapter in his book on children's diseases entitled 'Of Pyssing in the Bed', and 200 years later, in 1777, the appropriately named Dr Thomas Leake suggested an uncomfortable device to keep the sufferer awake so that he could not wet the bed in his sleep. At one time it was thought lucky if your urine dripped onto your toes. Urine was often used as an ingredient in medicines and was considered beneficial for corns and warts on the feet or as an application on sores and spots on the face. Fresh urine is mildly antiseptic, so this was not such a bad idea.

It was not until the nineteenth century that food and drink were recognized as having important effects on the bladder, including causing incontinence. Patients were advised, as they are today, to avoid tea and coffee. They were also told to cut out salt. It makes people thirsty so they drink more and so pass more water.

The patron saint of librarians, philosophers and sufferers from incontinence is St Catherine of Alexandria. Prayer to her is the treatment of last resort.

The sufferer of incontinence lives in constant dread of an 'accident' and when one does occur she or he (of the three million people affected in Britain the majority are women) makes haste to explain it away as though it had never happened before. She feels embarrassed, ashamed and helpless. Self-confidence drains to rock bottom and as for romance – forget it.

Every trip or visit is fraught with the fear that there won't be a handy loo, or that she won't be able to get there in time. She tries not to drink – tea, coffee, alcohol, anything liquid – until she feels uncomfortably dry. When she does succumb and has the longed-for

INTRODUCTION

cup of tea, she worries and wants to empty her bladder every five minutes – 'to be on the safe side'. It is humiliating to keep asking where the cloakroom is, and impossible to explain.

Big chunks of life and numerous fiddly details have to be organized round the facilities, for instance staying in an hotel or, even trickier, in a friend's house. None of this was a problem in the Middle Ages when most people slept on the floor on disposable bedding – straw – and the city streets were awash with human and animal excrement. Hygiene struck an all-time low and the stench was taken for granted – until nearly the end of the eighteenth century when Dr Leake's work came out.

This era saw a revolution in toilet engineering, with plumbing, sewage works and the introduction of the water closet on the practical side, while on the moral aspects John Wesley had already declared that 'cleanliness is next to godliness' (Sermons xciii). The Victorian outlook, redolent of prudery and guilt, ushered in the present-day secrecy and sense of shame attached to bodily functions below the waist – incontinence among them.

Sigmund Freud at the turn of the twentieth century pointed out that young children feel no instinctive disgust or guilt about these matters. It is something the grown-ups teach them. The cleanliness ethic flourishes still today in Europe and even more in the USA, witness the firms that have sprung up that will 'sell you a bathroom' as though it were something quite separate from the house or flat. But a state-of-the-art bathroom, jacuzzi and all, fades into insignificance compared with leak-proof efficiency in your personal plumbing.

With an ageing population more and more people are being made miserable by incontinence. It is estimated that it affects at least three million people in Britain, the majority of them women. The average-sized general practice carries some 5,500 patients with urinary incontinence, and around 900 who cannot control their motions – faecal incontinence. Twenty-five per cent of women over 40 suffer from some degree of incontinence compared with 3 per cent of men. Why the big difference? Women can have babies and their bodies are designed with this as top priority. By age 60, 40 per cent of women are incontinent, and nearly all of these have had children – the more kids the greater the risk.

There is no difficulty in talking about, say, arthritis or hiatus

INTRODUCTION

hernia, but although it causes immense distress, incontinence is never discussed openly. Instead it is concealed from friends, relatives, nearest and dearest – and the doctor. This means that sufferers get no sympathy and no support. One in three women, across the age spectrum from 15 upwards, 'leak' at least once in any one month. Forty per cent of those over 65 have to take regular precautions against leakages, such as pads or chair and mattress protectors, and frequent trips to the loo. Sixty per cent of the elderly who live in nursing homes are there because of incontinence rather than their other troubles.

It is often the final straw, the one disability that the most loving relative finds unacceptable.

If you ask someone old and hopefully wise what can be done about the problem, it's odds on they'll tell you that it is simply the price of motherhood and you just have to accept it. That is two myths in one sentence. First, there is plenty you can and should do to improve matters, and second, although having babies may cause temporary incontinence, it need not be a life sentence. Usually the situation recovers by itself within a few weeks. Treatment, including surgery, is available if necessary, while specific exercises are mandatory for all women after having a baby.

Before it develops into a nuisance, ordinary incontinence comes on very gradually, but even a single, small leak is immediately noticeable, and worrying to the sufferer. Apart from the elderly, it is particularly common among girls and women who are keen on healthy exercise – runners, tennis players, golfers and those doing power walking or aerobics. Leaks can be triggered by any strong or sudden muscular movement, including the involuntary contraction of the tummy muscles accompanying a cough or a sneeze. Anxiety on its own can also lead to leakage by tensing the muscles.

Since most women have an occasional leak it is useful to know what can be dismissed as normal and what requires attention.

These are OK:

- passing water 4–6 times a day
- passing water once (only) at night
- pants dry all through the day
- ability to 'hold on' without passing water for 3–5 hours
- no pain or strain on passing water

INTRODUCTION

- strong, continuous stream, not a hesitant dribble
- ability to stop and start in midstream if you choose

If you can put a tick to each of these, you have nothing to worry about. To stay this way, as you get older, is mainly a matter of a healthy lifestyle for your whole mind and body, including reasonable consideration for your waterworks – for instance, plenty of water to drink. Times to be extra thoughtful about this are during puberty, during pregnancy and the following six weeks, and through the menopause and the senior years.

The chances are that your urinary system will serve you well all your life, without any serious problems. However, if you notice the beginnings of a troublesome situation, you need to take action. This book helps you to choose the best ploys available – by one who knows from experience.

1
The waterworks – what they consist of and how they work

The organ that concerns us most is the *urinary* bladder – to distinguish it from, for instance, the gall bladder. The urinary bladder is basically a strong, stretchy bag that lies practically flat when it is empty, but becomes round as it fills with urine. It has a tough outer skin and a delicate lining like the inside of the mouth. Between these two layers is the *detrusor muscle*. Its fibres are so arranged that they contract simultaneously to expel all the urine that is in the bladder when the order comes from the brain.

The bladder lies in the *pelvis* – Greek for basin. It consists of a deep bony ring with a floor of fibre and muscle, lying at the bottom of the abdomen. It supports and partly encloses the pelvic organs. These comprise some concerned with reproduction, and some with the disposal of waste, both liquid, the urine, and solid, the motions. The arrangement is slightly different in the two sexes.

The bladder is at the centre of the pelvis, near the front, just behind the pubic symphysis. This is where the two pubic bones join together. You cannot feel your bladder except when it is full and rides up above the rim of the symphysis into the abdomen. If you press on it then, you get the urge to pass water. The other organs sharing the pelvis include the lower part of the colon, called the pelvic colon, and leading from that the rectum, which in turn leads into the anus or exit, via the short anal canal.

In men the sexual apparatus is outside, on display, but in women the pelvis provides a safe haven for such important sex organs as the vagina, the uterus (womb), the ovaries and the Fallopian tubes. A woman's pelvis is wider and shallower than a man's, a design that allows for the accommodation of these organs and also a foetus. Various pipes run through the pelvis – the two ureters, or urine tubes, each conveying fresh urine from the kidneys to the bladder; the Fallopian tubes, where egg and sperm meet, and the urethra, a canal conveying the urine from the bladder to the outside, for disposal.

The urethra is particularly short in women, 4 cm compared with the male 18–20 cm. This makes it vulnerable to infection from the outside world, or irritation from bubble baths and talcum powder. It has two sphincters, internal and external. These rings of muscle are the gate-keepers. They act like a drawstring to prevent the uncontrolled escape of urine from the bladder. The internal, or intrinsic, sphincter is sited in the urethral wall next to the external sphincter at the exit.

The membrane lining the sphincters, the trigone or triangle, is the most sensitive part of the bladder. Anything that irritates the bladder is felt most intensely here; it is the trigger point for passing water, voluntarily or otherwise.

The pelvic floor consists of a thin sheet of muscle and fibre. It not only helps to support the pelvic organs but backs up the action of the sphincters, especially in an emergency situation. It has quick-acting muscle fibres. However, its structure is weakened by the numerous tubes and vessels running through it and it can be over-stretched and damaged during childbirth. This is one of the contributory causes of stress incontinence in women.

Micturition

Micturition and urination are both Latin terms for the act of passing water – the procedure that is faulty in incontinence. Although it is so commonplace it is a complex action, involving precise co-ordination between different sets of nerves, the spinal cord and the brain. It works through several *reflexes*, those automatic responses to special triggers, like the involuntary jerk of your leg when the doctor taps it just below the kneecap.

The micturition reflex is more complicated than that, however. You first get an inkling that your bladder is getting full when it contains 175–250 ml of urine. This stretches the bladder wall slightly, setting off a reaction through the nerve endings it contains – advance information. If you do nothing the feeling gradually subsides, but returns more strongly when the volume of urine is over 350 ml, and urgently when it is nearing 500 ml. The absolute limit is somewhere between 500 and 800 ml, becoming less as you mature past 40. Gravity increases the pressure on the base of the bladder and the nerves in its wall flash a message to your brain that you must locate a loo – soon.

Meanwhile you can suppress, by your will, the reflex impulse to pass water. This is something you learned to do as a toddler, which cut down the 'puddle' rate dramatically. Starting the act of micturition is also something you learned young. You can choose when you want to do it. Most subtle of all, you are able to stop and start in midstream.

The bladder is filled continuously from the kidneys, through the ureters. The sphincters that close off your bladder remain tight shut until you decide that the time and place are convenient for passing the collected urine. The sphincters and the pelvic floor muscles then relax and another reflex comes into play. This tells the detrusor muscle to contract, and empty the bladder.

The muscles that are under the control of the will are the detrusor, the sphincter muscles and those of the pelvic floor. The last are weaker than the others, and work at a disadvantage because they are unsupported and together with the accompanying ligaments come under strain during a difficult birth.

The automatic rescue package

Have you ever heard anyone say: 'It was so funny I nearly wet myself laughing'? It is no joke when it happens. When you get a sudden impulse to cough, sneeze or laugh, or you lift something heavy, the pressure inside your abdomen, including your bladder, shoots up. It can overwhelm your normal anti-flood defences, but fortunately the emergency service usually kicks in on time. Through its continuous monitoring of your body the autonomic, unconscious nervous system 'knows' a split second in advance that you are about to sneeze or whatever. Immediately, a reflex message shoots down the nerves to cut short the action of the detrusor (emptying) muscle. The bladder relaxes and the quick-acting pelvic floor muscles, followed by the sphincters, close the exit. The day is saved!

The pelvic floor

The pelvic floor muscles are versatile and constantly useful. The most important of them is the *pubococcygeus*, running from the pubic bones at the front to the *coccyx*, the rudimentary tail at the base of the spine. Their general role is to support the pelvic organs and help the sphincters to prevent leakages. Although they come under voluntary control, the knack of controlling the pelvic floor muscles is often poorly mastered. Urination itself is less well controlled, particularly in women. Mothers, with the best intentions, sometimes teach their children faulty urinating patterns, that it is best to 'go' when you don't need to because it is convenient (see p. 113).

Girls should learn to recognize the feeling of contracting and relaxing the pelvic floor muscles and gain some control over them. The tension in these muscles is responsible for sexual arousal and orgasm, and also stimulates lubrication in the area.

In the less developed countries girls at puberty, those getting married and starting sexual intercourse, and women in the weeks after having a baby, are taught pelvic floor exercises. The squatting position, so natural in Asia and Africa, exercises and strengthens the pelvic floor. Women in these areas seldom suffer from incontinence.

If the pelvic floor muscles are weak for any reason, intercourse cannot reach the peak of pleasure, and in childbirth the mother is unable to work effectively. Incontinence afterwards is more likely and another result may be prolapse (see Chapter 8).

It is surprising that such a delicately balanced procedure as passing water does not go wrong more often. A leakage is always disconcerting to the sufferer, and to make matters worse other people simply do not understand. Because it most often happens to oldies, others are apt to confuse a problem in the plumbing with senility and brain failure. This is incorrect and upsetting. Those who suffer from leakages include men, women and children of all ages, some more vulnerable than others.

Sufferers from leakages, in order of prevalence, are:

1 *Women*, especially mothers of 45-plus with several children.
2 *Men* of 60–70. Their problems peak when their prostate gland, situated at the base of the bladder, enlarges, blocking the outflow. This is an age-related event.
3 *Children* who are slow to acquire the knack of dryness or who have slipped back into baby ways later – often because of some emotional trauma. Divorce at home or bullying at school are frequent causes.
4 *Adolescents*, whose hormonal upheaval, and for girls the start of their periods, makes for a general excitability of the pelvic organs.

THE WATERWORKS

5 *Older men and women*, whose muscles, including the detrusor, the sphincters and those of the pelvic floor, are less strong, have weaker bladder control.
6 *Frail old people* may lose their nervous control of urination. Messages fail to get through and the bladder lets urine dribble out continuously, or floods without warning.

2
The big problem

The top problem with the waterworks is a plumbing failure – leakiness. It comes in several different varieties. *Stress incontinence* is the commonest type, accounting for 50 per cent of cases. It is basically due to weakness of the urethral sphincters, the muscular door-keepers of the exit from the bladder, together with their little helpers, the muscles of the pelvic floor. *Urge incontinence* – you can't wait – is due to bladder instability and accounts for another 15 per cent of sufferers. The rest are made up of a combination of these two conditions, and some others, such as obstruction or nerve damage.

Stress incontinence

This is almost universal among women at some time in their lives. The exact numbers are not known because so many suffer in secret. Men are scarcely affected at all because of their convenient anatomy, whereas gravity is constantly adding to the pressure on a girl's or a woman's pelvic organs. Stress incontinence can affect people of any age, including children, but like all water problems, it tends to get worse when you pass 40.

It occurs when there is an upsurge of pressure inside the abdomen, automatically involving the bladder. If it is intense or sudden it may catch the anti-leakage mechanism by surprise. The leak is usually small, but it can loose a flood. Any active sport, lifting something heavy – or even just touching your toes – will increase the pressure, while trivial matters like coughing, sneezing or giggling have a brief but powerful effect.

The root of the problem is muscle weakness. This is likely to result from overstretching of the muscle fibres during a long or difficult labour – or twins! Normal ageing from the mid forties onwards leads to weakening of the muscles all over the body including the sphincters. The pressure inside the bladder increases as its capacity shrinks progressively over the years, while the volume of urine remains the same. As the menopause approaches there is also a lessening in the supportive role of the sex hormones to all the tissues. Another sign of stress incontinence apart from leaking is a weak stream, degenerating into a dribble.

Physical damage to the urethra, especially the sphincter, can be the cause of stress incontinence in men. It sometimes happens in the course of TURP (transurethral prostatectomy), an operation to remove the prostate performed through the penis.

Patricia
Patricia was a cigarette addict and when she developed bronchitis on top of her smoker's tickle, she went through paroxysms of coughing. They made her eyes run – and her bladder leak. The combined efforts of the sphincter and the pelvic floor could not withstand the pressure. The situation was ruining Patricia's life, so after years of smoking she was finally sufficiently motivated to give it up. This was a start on her route to urinary control. She is now working at pelvic floor exercises.

Urgency and urge incontinence

Urgency comprises such a powerful impulse to pass water that you feel you will never be able to resist it before you get to the loo. Sometimes you can regain control temporarily, and struggle the distance cross-legged, but you may not manage it. Urge and stress incontinence can, and often do, occur together and are sometimes complicated by frequency. However, they have different causes and need different treatment. While a weak sphincter is the underlying fault in stress incontinence, urgency usually results from a bladder that contracts inconsistently.

Rosemary
Rosemary, 65, had a large-scale map of Guildford, her home town, with the public and other available toilets highlighted because of her frequency – coupled with urgency. She had no sooner emptied her bladder at one facility than she was looking for another, and she could never sit right through a theatre performance. Her friends teased her about it, but her husband

found it tiresome. Finally she undertook a course of training in bladder control which helped after two months of effort.

Urgency comes in two types – *sensory* and *motor*.

Sensory urgency

Sensory urgency is a matter of feeling or sensation, and occurs when the bladder is inflamed or irritated, for instance by an infection, a stone or a tumour. Usually the feeling can be controlled and accidental leakage is avoided. A special form occurs in adolescent girls, *giggle micturition* or *enuresis risoria*. Other intense emotional states may also be responsible.

Motor urgency

Motor urgency, in contrast to sensory urgency, nearly always leads to incontinence. It is the result of *bladder instability*, with the unpredictable action of the detrusor, the main muscle for emptying the bladder. It may begin contracting irregularly while the bladder is still only half empty, and it is out of phase with the muscles of the sphincter. This is known as *dyssynergia*. As with most types of incontinence, women are more susceptible than men and often the simple action of standing up, bringing gravity into play, is enough to trigger a leak. Treatment is aimed at relaxing the detrusor and medication is usually helpful.

Urge incontinence in women is usually *idiopathic*, a long word for saying we don't know the cause. It may be idiopathic in men too, but in them it is more often associated with obstruction to the outflow of urine by an enlarged prostate.

Overflow incontinence

This is characterized by a continuous dribble of urine or a series of small leaks with any muscular effort. There are two basic types, according to their cause – physical obstruction to the outflow of urine or loss of nervous control of the emptying process. In the first type the urine escapes round the edges of the blockage. Obstruction is a fairly common problem in a man, due to an enlarged prostate, but it can occur very occasionally in a woman with a pregnant uterus.

In the type due to loss of nervous control there is inefficient emptying of the bladder so that it is permanently part full, and simply overflows like any other vessel. The causes include stroke, multiple sclerosis, diabetic neuropathy and Parkinsonism.

The sufferers of both types are constantly wet, but especially in those with nerve impairment, chronic infection is common in the stagnant urine.

Stephen
Stephen was 70 when he started finding his underwear wet every evening and gradually all day, too. His wife thought he was getting old and careless, and he felt helpless. He was also troubled by not being able to pass water when he wanted, but having to wait a few frustrating moments before a weak stream dribbled out. His doctor soon diagnosed the problem – an enlarged prostate. Stephen was cured by a quickie operation via the penis.

Continuous or total incontinence

Occasionally a false passage, called a fistula, may develop between the bladder and the vagina or the uterus after radiotherapy or as an accidental result of surgery. Serious damage to the spinal cord or congenital abnormality are other possible causes. The sufferer has no control over the bladder. An operation is the only possible help.

Reflex incontinence

This form is seen in paraplegics, in whom the connections from the brain are interrupted. It usually requires long-term catheterization.

Age-related incontinence

This is very common, since we all grow older. It is usually first noticeable as a mild tendency to 'a weak bladder' at around 40, gradually increasing through the climacteric years, as the ovaries retire. In men there may be a midlife crisis at this time. The slow progression continues through the sixties, then the third and fourth ages into grand old age. You are expected to make less and less physical effort at home or work, so you require less muscle power. Your muscles shrink and lose their power, including those of the urinary apparatus. Strangely, the bowel retains more of its strength than the waterworks do, but both systems become less efficient together with the abdominal muscles. You cannot help losing your figure as the abdominal muscles slacken.

Anal and double incontinence

When nervous control fails and particularly when the anal sphincter, analogous to the urinary sphincters, has become slack and weak, a frail elderly person may become *doubly incontinent* and lose control over passing motions as well as water.

Pseudo-incontinence

This variety, in contrast to many of the others, always has a definite cause outside the urinary system, rather than a physical fault within it.

Common underlying conditions include:

- Persistent cough, asthma and smoking.
- Following a bout of pneumonia.
- Chronic constipation with straining by the muscles of the abdomen to overcome it.
- Infection not only of the bladder, cystitis, but of the colon or other pelvic organs. This makes the bladder irritable and brings on frequency. Passing water may be excruciatingly painful.
- Water tablets, diuretics, given for swelling ankles, high blood pressure and heart problems, may be too effective so that you have to pass water when you do not wish to. If the diuretic is taken first thing, when your joints may be stiff, this increases the risk of not reaching the toilet in time.
- Some antidepressants have diuretic side-effects.
- Sleeping tablets may work too strongly and prevent you waking up when your bladder needs relieving.
- Caffeine, especially in percolated coffee, but also in tea and cola drinks, irritates the bladder muscles causing urgency and frequency.

THE BIG PROBLEM

- The alpha-blocker group of drugs for high blood pressure and heart failure, for instance Hypovase (prazosin), interfere with the action of the pelvic floor muscles, the bladder itself and in particular the sphincter.
- Alcohol has a double effect. It inflames your bladder and, in a big dose, fuddles your brain, clouding body awareness and muscle co-ordination. It transfers water from the tissues to the kidneys, setting up a thirst.
- Disc and spinal problems may cause paralysis of the pelvic floor muscles.
- You may have reasonably good bladder control but may not be able to get to the toilet in time because of arthritis, an injury or Parkinson's disease.
- Pregnancy, especially in weeks 10–12 and in the last month.
- During the recovery period after having a baby or an abdominal operation such as the removal of an ovary.
- The progressive brain diseases like Alzheimer's or Parkinson's disease in which you gradually lose control of your body as well as your mind, and brain damage from stroke or tumour.
- Confusion when you wake up in the night, especially in a strange place, as when on holiday, or when you have an infection – chest or waterworks.

What to do when you find you are having problems with your water

First and most important is frank and open discussion with your doctor, and co-operation with her or him to pinpoint the cause. Get all the information you can, since this is likely to be a long-lasting or recurrent problem and it helps to understand it.

Quick identifier of your type of incontinence

Type	Stress	Urge	Overflow	Continuous
Symptoms	leak with raised pressure	urgency, frequency	hesitancy, poor stream, incomplete emptying, frequency	unaware of leak
Size of leak	small	may be great	small	inconspicuous

Now come the ploys for dealing with the situation. Above all, whichever type of incontinence you have, be prepared to follow patiently the advice on lifestyle, especially on exercise. It *will* help.

3
The middle years

The two decades of age 35–55 are a second adolescence. The first time round you were a budding then a blossoming teenager. It was a period of tremendous, exciting change. Hormones that had lain dormant sprang into life. You were transformed from a child into an adult capable of being a mother, or father, reaching your full height, and with muscle power increasing to full strength.

It was at this time, when all these things were happening, that women will have had their *menarche* (*men* means monthly), the start of what is popularly known as the curse. This is the four-weekly bleed that follows the shedding of an egg-cell that has not been fertilized. The body is geared up for having babies, and feeding them. From around 15 an occasional blip with loss of control of the water is not uncommon – a leak brought on by running, sneezing, coughing or the giggles – stress incontinence.

The climacteric or perimenopause

The second adolescence, the *climacteric* in women, is also a time of hormonal upheaval with great mental and physical changes. These are to fit you for the next important stage of life – *mature adulthood*. Now you want your body to run efficiently and economically, and you can dispense with 'the curse' and the milk-making apparatus.

The term *climacteric* comes from climax, the Greek word for a ladder or stepwise progression, while an alternative term, the *perimenopause*, comes from both Greek and Latin, *peri* meaning around. This time it consists of a series of physiological changes, working towards the menopause over several years, with continuing adjustments for a further few years afterwards. The whole process can drag on for as long as 20 years altogether, or be completed in as little as five. Some women are plagued by a mixed bag of symptoms throughout, while others sail through with hardly any inconvenience. Most are somewhere between.

Since the waterworks and the sexual organs are so intimately involved, it is no wonder that during the ongoing disturbance of the climacteric, problems with the water, specifically incontinence, are likely to arise. Special risk factors are emotional stress, especially involving anxiety, or a recent hysterectomy. Fifty per cent have water problems for several months after the operation.

The menopause

This, unlike the climacteric, is a single discrete event on a particular day – the last day of your very last period. You can only pinpoint it in retrospect – after a year with no bleeds. Today we live longer and the menopause comes later. The average age for it now, in the twenty-first century, is 50 years and 9 months, compared with just 50 in the mid twentieth century. While the menopause used to signal the end of our youth, now we have around 40 good years of life ahead of us. Dickens, in the mid nineteenth century, wrote of an 'old man' of 50. At that time the expectation of life was only 45 for a woman because of the dangers of childbirth; now we can expect to flourish well into our eighties. The post-menopausal stage covers an enormous slice of our life.

The periods, or menses, run in a hormonally controlled cycle of ovulation (the release of an egg), the breakdown of the lining of the womb (the bleed), and then its rebuilding.

The underlying force for all this comes from the pinhead-sized ovum, or egg-cell, and the hormones it produces. It is when the monthly release of egg-cells falters, finally to stop, that the unobtrusive changes of the climacteric – such as slight thinning of the hair – get under way and merge with the more obvious and less desirable 'menopausal symptoms'. They are all due to a shortage of the chief female hormone, oestrogen, and are at their most troublesome when there is a fluctuant situation and your body is deprived of the hormone at one time and has plenty at another.

Other factors affecting the supply of oestrogen

- *Mood and emotion* – warm, happy feelings encourage production while stress and unhappiness reduce it.
- *Too much or too little thyroid hormone* – either may interfere with making oestrogen.
- *Diet* – slimmers and anorexics and others who are underweight

tend to have low levels of oestrogen while plump people can make all they need.

What oestrogen does for you

- Stimulates your sexual development at puberty.
- Maintains the structure of the breasts, uterus and vagina and also of the urethra (urine tube) and the sensitive area, the trigone, at the base of the bladder.
- Stimulates the lubrication of the vagina and the production of collagen which supports the skin, keeping wrinkles at bay.
- Slows down the thinning and dryness of the skin and hair which occurs with the passing years.
- Helps the bones to take up calcium, protecting them against osteoporosis.
- Maintains the smoothness of the joint surfaces, delaying the development of the wear-and-tear disorder, osteoarthritis.
- Checks the amount of fat in the blood, helping to prevent blocked arteries and coronary attacks.
- Retains the elasticity of the blood vessels, allowing them to carry, in the blood, the maximum amount of oxygen to the tissues, including the brain.
- Tends to increase the amount of protein in the body, but it is male hormone that is needed to help muscle building.
- Last but not least, oestrogen supports both mental and physical energy and a stable, generally hopeful mood.

Alternative sources of oestrogen

Since oestrogen is so important, when the main supply dwindles as egg production is cut, your body draws what it can from other sources. The ovaries continue to make a little for some years after the periods have finished, and some of the testosterone converts to oestrogen. The adrenal glands (*ad* means near, *renal* kidney) are now the main manufacturers of the hormone and they increase production as the need is felt. Spare body fat is used to make a weak form of oestrogen called *oestrone* and it is noticeable that many plump women sail through the menopause with no signs of oestrogen deficiency. An extra bonus is their youthful-looking complexion.

Phyto-oestrogens are another group of weak oestrogens. They are derived from plants and good sources include soya, tofu, ginseng, alfalfa, green and yellow vegetables, rhubarb, celery, liquorice, almonds, mung beans, black cohosh and aniseed.

The other sex hormones

Progesterone, like oestrogen, is made in the ovaries, but in decreasing amounts as ovulation becomes less frequent. It is far less important than oestrogen, but a shortage of it leads to heavy, unpredictable periods.

Testosterone, the male hormone, is also produced in the ovaries in small quantities. This increases after the menopause and may cause a slight increase in facial hair. It is also responsible for libido, the drive towards sex.

Early effects of lack of oestrogen

These effects arise in the run-up to the menopause and continue into the months or years following it. There is a general shrinkage of the genital and urinary organs, which are close neighbours, accompanied by the following indications:

- blood flow to them is reduced
- lubrication is lessened, making them drier
- collagen packing tissue is reduced, making the skin and membranes thinner and more fragile – and with more lines
- increased local susceptibility to infection
- loss of pubic hair
- disrupted periods – early or late or wildly unpredictable, and extra heavy or very light. The trend is towards wider spacing and diminishing blood loss.

Vasomotor symptoms

Vasomotor symptoms are the commonest cause of discomfort in the perimenopause. *Vaso* refers to the blood vessels, *motor* means movement. The only movements blood vessels can make are dilating and constricting, letting more or less blood through, most noticeably to the skin, which can look ashy pale or scarlet. The key vasomotor symptoms are:

- hot flushes
- night sweats
- palpitations

Hot flushes

Hot flushes are uncomfortable and often embarrassingly visible. They come in waves lasting a matter of seconds up to 15 minutes. First is a feeling of pressure in your head as the small blood vessels open up, then the skin rapidly becomes lobster red and feels hot. This usually starts in the neck, and spreads upwards involving your face to the roots of your hair and sometimes extending to your chest and shoulders. Eventually your whole body may be involved. Sweating, a thumping heartbeat and a sense of panic can all be part of the picture. You may have hot flushes several times a day, and in a third of women the flushes continue sporadically for as long as five years.

> *Alice*
> Alice was a fair-skinned blonde. When she was 46 she began blushing brick red, as she had as a teenager, but with different stimuli. Then it was a response to embarrassing social situations, but now the main triggers were tea or coffee, a hot curry, an overheated room or exercise. Apart from avoiding these, the most effective management was HRT, hormone replacement therapy, in which the chief ingredient is oestrogen.

Night sweats

Night sweats may wake you up in the small hours drenched with hot or cold sweat, accompanied by a racing heart. The sweats tend to follow the same time-scale as the flushes, building up to a crescendo then tailing off some time after the actual menopause.

Palpitations

Palpitations occur when the opening up of the blood vessels automatically involves a quickening of the heart rate which is unpleasantly obvious to the sufferer. You may feel faint and generally weak and shaky.

Other symptoms often ascribed to the menopause include head, neck and backache, poor sleep, weight gain, sore breasts, bloating and fatigue without any cause. Added to all these pinpricks of misery there is, for many of us, the horrid surprise of finding we sometimes have wet pants or an ominous warm trickle down the thigh – incontinence. The cause may be understandable, for instance not getting to the loo quickly enough because, say, you have injured your ankle. Usually the reason is not so obvious.

Your waterworks are closely involved with the sexual system, and the mucous membrane lining the bladder and urethra is affected similarly to that in the vagina and uterus by the shortage of oestrogen.

Vaginitis

Vaginitis is inflammation and soreness of the vagina when the lining becomes thinner, dryer and more delicate as its supply of oestrogen is diminished. It may feel generally sore, and painful during sexual intercourse – *dyspareunia*. It may even bleed a little.

At the same time, the lining of the trigone, the doorkeeper to the bladder, like the lining of the vagina, becomes thin and extra sensitive as the lack of oestrogen takes effect. This triggers a frequent impulse to pass water and often causes urge incontinence.

Erica

Erica was lucky. She had been widowed for three years and was 57 when she met Harry. He was just 60. He fell for her bright good looks and happy nature and since there seemed no reason to delay they were married within three months. The honeymoon, in Venice, was a disaster. Erica had had no sexual activity for seven years, since her late husband was not well enough in his final, drawn-out illness. She had not even indulged in masturbation, which would have helped with her sexual response and lubrication.

As it was, what should have been an adult pleasure turned out to be a painful experience which she could not face repeating without some relief. KY jelly, liberally applied, was a first-line help, but even more effective was the dienoestrol ointment. This local application replaced the oestrogen she was lacking from her own resources. Her occasional leakage of urine also improved when the vaginitis no longer made the area so sensitive.

Cystitis

As the bladder lining becomes thinner and more liable to break down infection easily sets in – cystitis. More than 10 per cent of women over 60 are currently suffering from cystitis and nearly all of us fall victim to it at least once in our lives (see Chapter 17).

Later – long-term effects of lack of oestrogen

- Osteoporosis – women run ten times the risk of men.
- Furred-up arteries due to upset fat metabolism, increasing the risk of stroke, coronary artery disease and high blood pressure.
- Shortage of collagen leading to thinning and weakening of skin, membranes, muscles and joint surfaces.
- Slow healing, for instance with varicose ulcers.

Olivia
Olivia was 60 when free bone densitometry tests were offered at her local health centre. Bone densitometry measures by X-ray the strength and solidity of the bones, and is a diagnostic test for the risk of osteoporosis. Olivia was shocked to find that she was well into the risk area, although she had taken regular exercise for years, with supplements of calcium and a range of vitamins including vitamin D (calciferol). She ate plenty of cheese, sardines and yoghurt, containing both calcium and calciferol, but she was a heavy tea-drinker and the caffeine would have inhibited the absorption of the calcium. Also, she often took a dose of indigestion mixture, the aluminium-based type, which had a similar effect.

Following her doctor's advice Olivia changed to a non-aluminium indigestion mixture and *scrupulously avoided tea, coffee and chocolate drinks*. The serendipitous bonus was that she was relieved of the symptoms she had never mentioned to her doctor – her frequency and urge incontinence. They had been caused by the seven or eight cups of strong, caffeine-laden tea she drank as a matter of habit every day.

4
The male angle

Although women are far more often the sufferers of genitourinary problems – sex, reproduction and waterworks – men are not immune. For women, it is in the middle years, especially from 50 onwards, that problems arise, including incontinence. It is the physical legacy of bearing children and the dwindling supply of oestrogen as the ovaries pack up that lead to the symptoms.

Midlife is a dodgy time for men, too, just when they feel they should be at their peak, career-wise, physically and sexually. But, as for their female partners, it turns out to be the age when health problems begin to show their teeth. Not big, life-threatening events but embarrassing difficulties with urination, a disconcerting unpredictability over erections, and the beginnings of a pot belly. These developments do nothing for a man's self-confidence.

While many women have endless troubles with the menopause and their ability to procreate wanes away, men remain fertile indefinitely but their sexual performance falls off. Health journalists and doctors, the editors of women's magazines and women themselves, endlessly analyse the changes that beset menopausal women. This is in sharp contrast to the paucity of literature about the 50-plus male.

It is time for the spotlight to illumine the bodily and psychological revolution that engulfs men of equivalent age. Men themselves need to be aware of what to expect, and so too do those who have charge of them, usually their wives.

The *andropause* or *viropause* (Greek or Latin) is where the suffering menopausal female gets the last laugh. The organ responsible is a small gland that has been of no account in the man's first half-century but is at the centre of his problems in the second. Where for women it is the ovaries, womb and vagina that show their age, in men it is the prostate alone that evens up the disparity between the sexes for unwelcome symptoms of middle age, including urinary incontinence.

One task of the prostate is to produce the nourishing fluid that feeds the sperm on its marathon swim to reach the ovum, but its other functions are uncertain.

Disorders of the prostate

Any of the following may be associated with incontinence.

- benign hyperplasia
- prostatitis – inflammation with or without infection
- prostadynia – a bundle of symptoms related to the prostate, but with no discoverable cause
- prostate cancer

Benign hyperplasia

This is an extremely common condition in man and one other creature, his faithful hound. *Hyper* means over, and *plasia* growth, and benign means there is nothing cancerous about it. A young, healthy prostate is around the size of a walnut, but unlike the general shrinkage of the female sex and water apparatus, the prostate gets bigger with age, reaching the size of an apricot. This begins from around age 40 and by 60, 50 per cent of men have an enlarged prostate, escalating to 90 per cent by age 80.

Hyperplasia would not matter if it were not for the position of the gland. It hugs the urethra close to the sphincter and as it gets bigger it puts the squeeze on the outflow of urine. The bladder becomes overfull and the muscle fibres and nerve endings in its walls are stretched. The pressure on the latter causes the 'can't wait' syndrome, resulting in urge incontinence.

Prostatism

Prostatism is the name given to the complex of symptoms associated with an enlarged prostate. They include:

- getting up to pass water more than once in the night
- frequent trips to the loo in the day
- slow, weak stream
- incomplete emptying
- a sense of urgency but when the chap arrives at the loo he may have to wait for agonizing moments before the flow starts

- dribbling towards the end of the act. In conjunction with the weak stream, this accounts for the familiar 'spill' stains round the base of men's toilets.

If he has these symptoms there is a 90 to 1 likelihood that the poor fellow has benign hyperplasia, but it is vital and may be life-saving for his doctor to check him out for a urinary infection or the big baddie, prostate cancer. In other cases, there may be conditions outside the waterworks such as anxiety, which can disturb a man's sleep. If he wakes in the night, whatever the reason, he may automatically feel he must pass water – this is not frequency.

> *Gerald*
> Gerald, nudging 60, was unaware of his large prostate until after a good but not excessive dinner with wine. He suddenly found he could not relieve himself although he desperately wanted to. He was in increasingly acute distress until a doctor passed a catheter into his bladder, releasing Niagara. Gerald was suffering from *acute retention*. After this alarming experience he was only too glad to be rid of the rogue organ and followed his doctor's advice to have a prostatectomy, surgical removal of the gland.

There are other ploys for less extreme symptoms.

Treatment
The symptoms, not the size of the prostate, dictate the management of hyperplasia. Only one in four men with prostatism actually need medical help. Mild symptoms may only require the cutting down or avoidance of the food and drink known to inflame the urinary system. Alcohol comes high on the list of irritants.

There are several herbal remedies that may help and do no harm. Saw palmetto is a favourite with the Americans, and others are horsetail, pumpkin seeds, goldenrod and pulsatilla, as tea or tablets. Dietary recommendations include vitamins D and E, and plenty of fibre, folic acid and beta-carotene – in green and yellow vegetables.

Of the straight pharmaceuticals, the alpha-blocker finasteride (Proscar) at a dosage of one 5 mg tablet daily is one of the best. It needs to be taken for at least six months to assess its effectiveness, and continued indefinitely if the results are favourable. It acts by relaxing the muscle fibres in the gland, helping to improve the feeble flow of urine through the tense, thickened tissues. The feeling of incomplete emptying is lessened, also the need to pass water several times at night. The progression of the disorder is slowed down, delaying the need for an operation or avoiding it altogether. Disappointingly, the side-effects may include loss of libido and impotence as well as dizziness and weakness.

The standard operation for removing the prostate is TURP – transurethral resection of the prostate. As the name suggests, the instruments are introduced through the urethra. There are several refinements available. Instead of a lancet, the surgeon may use diathermy (burning with an electric current), a laser, or a form of microwave. TUNA is nothing fishy but stands for *transurethral needle ablation* – destroying the prostate with radiowaves.

Prostatitis

Before age 40 prostate problems are a rarity, except for prostatitis.

Acute bacterial prostatitis is an infection with similar symptoms to those of cystitis – a burning sensation on passing water, urgency with a high risk of incontinence and frequency. There is lower back pain rather than in the abdomen as it is in cystitis; a raised temperature; delay in starting urination; and malaise, a feeling of illness. Antibiotics help, but the infection is often persistent and several courses may be needed.

Nonbacterial prostatitis resembles the bacterial type, but is milder and there is no obvious germ to blame. Is some undiscovered organism responsible, or an odd psychological quirk?

Prostadynia

In prostadynia all the tests score normal and nothing shows up on examination of the urinary system but the symptoms of prostatitis persist.

There is no essential difference between non-bacterial prostatitis and prostadynia and the only treatment is to avoid the usual suspects in urinary disorders – caffeine in all its guises, aspartame, spicy food, and alcohol. Some people advise avoiding salami, chilli and garlic.

THE MALE ANGLE
Prostate cancer

This common cancer is on the increase by 3 per cent per year, and is now the second commonest cause of death for men in the Western world. It is no respecter of people and sufferers include Ayatollah Khomeini, François Mitterrand, General Schwarzkopf, Bob Dole and Roger Moore. While women have a common enemy in breast cancer, men have prostate cancer. Breast cancer affects one in ten women, and there is a great deal of publicity about it. Prostate cancer gets one in 11 men but does not arouse such attention.

The symptoms may be just like those of benign hyperplasia, creeping on insidiously, but sometimes there is a warning with blood in the urine, at the beginning of the stream. In other cases, by contrast, the cancer goes unnoticed until secondaries are causing bone pain or the anaemia of chronic disease. We know a good deal about the risks. Some are unavoidable, for instance age. At 75-plus, 9 per cent of men have prostate cancer, escalating with every year. Having a first-degree relative (father, brother, grandfather) with the disease increases the risk two or three times, and black Americans run twice the risk of whites.

Environment, diet and lifestyle are important influences. The Western way of life increases the risks – for immigrants, including the Chinese, as well as natural-born Westerners. By contrast, Chinese men living in China have one of the lowest rates. The dangerous aspects of living in the First World in relation to prostate cancer are not smoking, drinking or drugs, but diet. Helpful items are the antioxidants, especially lycopene in cooked tomatoes, watermelon and pink grapefruit, betacarotene in carrots, folic acid in green vegetables and fibre from fruit and vegetables. Low-dose vitamin D also has a protective effect.

Screening is a must to 'catch' the cancer at the first suspicious symptom. The investigation is sure to include a digital (finger) examination of the gland via the back passage. No one likes that, and a new blood test may replace it.

Protein-specific antigen (PSA) estimation
PSA is an enzyme produced by all prostate tissue, whether or not it is cancerous, but a high level in the blood suggests malignant disease. An average reading is 4 ng/ml or less but with 4–10 ng/ml

there is nothing to distinguish cancer from benign hyperplasia. The normal level increases with age:

- age 40–49 – 2.5 ng/ml
- age 50–59 – 3.5 ng/ml
- age 60–69 – 4.5 ng/ml
- age 70–79 – 6.5 ng/ml

Levels significantly higher call for further investigation, first digitally, then with ultrasound and ultimately biopsy. Biopsy means taking a tiny sample of prostate tissue and examining it under the microscope to check the diagnosis.

Factors apart from age affecting the PSA results are:

- prostatitis
- prostate cancer
- catheterization
- biopsy procedure
- prostatectomy – surgical removal of the gland

Treatment of prostate cancer

The good news is that this disease is no longer the quick and certain killer it was a few years ago. For the older man, when his symptoms are slight, and the tumour is doing little but tick over, many physicians pursue a 'wait-and-see' policy. They do not intervene unless a problem arises. It is for the younger man – 65 or under – that active treatment is required. The choice lies between radiotherapy, cryotherapy (freezing), surgery and, for advanced disease, hormone therapy. A vaccine is also being developed.

Each method carries its own risks and benefits. For example, hormone treatment is not painful or even uncomfortable, but tends to have a feminizing effect, including impotence and slight breast development. The most favoured treatment is surgery, but there is a small risk of the two most feared side-effects – long-term impotence and incontinence. A new American device is said to warn the surgeon if he is in danger of injuring a vital nerve. Radiotherapy is most frequently called into play when surgery is not feasible or has failed. It douses out pain but the sufferer feels nauseous and exhausted for a day or two after each session.

THE MALE ANGLE

Urinary retention

Acute urinary retention

This is the disaster that befell Gerald. It crops up suddenly, although with hindsight there were probably warnings, such as sporadic hesitancy. The bladder may be full to bursting but the sufferer cannot make the sphincter relax for water to pass in the normal way. The likeliest cause is benign prostatic hypertrophy, but other possibilities must be considered:

- Prostate cancer.
- Stricture – a scarred or constricted place in the urethra, sometimes caused by the faulty passage of a catheter.
- Infection in the urinary tract, especially urethritis, with swelling blocking this narrow tube. Women very occasionally have acute retention from this cause.
- Rock-like constipation producing pressure through the rectum.
- Reaction to recent surgery in the pelvis.

There have usually been previous symptoms of threatened or mild obstruction. These include a poor, hesitant flow, petering out at the end of the act; intermittent symptoms; and *pis-en-deux*, which means literally 'pissing twice'. The bladder does not feel empty after passing water and there is an urge to try again immediately. There may be overflow incontinence.

The urgent treatment for acute retention is to pass a catheter up the urethra. If this is not possible because of a stricture or scarring from an earlier injury to the urethra, the catheter must be introduced suprapubically, that is through the abdomen, above the pubic symphysis. The prostate will be removed later.

Chronic retention

This is relatively commonplace. The bladder is always more or less full and often leaks – overflow incontinence – all the time or when there is extra pressure on it.

A rectal examination with the doctor's finger in the back passage and his other hand on the abdomen enables him or her to assess the size of the prostate and also to feel whether it has a smooth surface as in benign hyperplasia or craggy as in cancer. The strength of the anal sphincter can also be estimated – relevant to some cases of incontinence.

Dyssynergia of the neck of the bladder is a condition only seen in young and middle-aged men. It means a lack of concordance between the urinary sphincter and the detrusor muscle. Either incontinence or retention may result.

Stricture of the urethra, another cause of retention, may be due to accidental trauma or a sexually transmitted disorder (STD), but often has no discernible cause.

5
Juniors

We all start life incontinent, both for motions and water, and are blissfully unaware. The nerve pathways and reflexes that make up the control system are not yet complete. As with all of nature, each individual, whether flower or bird or baby, grows and develops at his or her own pace and there is nothing you can do to alter it.

You are bound to hear about someone else's baby who was clean and dry at a few months. This does not mean he was a wonder child or that his mother applied some marvellous training programme. It only means that this little one happened to pass his motion, with urine, at much the same time every day, and his vigilant mother learned to 'catch' it in the potty more often than not. The age at which a baby learns to use a potty is notorious for being the subject of more exaggeration than any other achievement.

In fact it is pointless and often counter-productive to start training too soon, that is before your child is even properly aware of what is happening below. It is usually when he is between 20 months and two years, after he has learned to walk, albeit in a wide-based waddle, that your toddler will show that he realizes that the puddle on the floor is due to him. This is the signal that his nervous system is now geared up to learn bladder and bowel control. He clinches the matter by inventing or adopting words for each function. These will be incorporated into the family language. They are likely to be simple, single-syllable words such as loo, poo, pee and wee.

Your role as a parent during these exciting developments is to inculcate a relaxed attitude about the whole matter, with the gentlest of encouragement. Grannies, usually such a reliable source of wisdom and support, are apt to be too concerned over toilet training. They often see it in terms of good and naughty or success and failure, and are best not involved. One mistake the young learners often make is to wet a clean, dry nappy as soon as it is put on. This is not thoughtless or done to annoy – it shows that baby has worked out what a nappy is for and to use it seems perfectly reasonable.

There are no hard and fast rules about what is normal progress in the long struggle against baby incontinence. Each toddler develops to his own rhythm, but masters control of the motions first, usually at around two. Between two and two-and-a-half he is learning to be dry in the day, and can manage most nights by the time he is three to three-and-a-half. However, these are only averages and a lot of nursery school youngsters do not achieve this until they are five, while 10 per cent don't get the knack of controlling their water before they are seven.

Between the ages of three and four your child grows two-and-a-half to 3 inches in height and acquires skills in jumping, running, climbing and throwing. Mentally he is learning to think, reason and use his imagination creatively. He feeds himself with knife, fork and spoon, and practises the most social skill of all – going to the loo on his own. By age four he will be a chatterbox and want to do everything 'by the self'. He is likely to need practice at home with wiping his own bottom. The new moist toilet paper makes this easier. Clothes tend to be bundled, rather than tucked in at the waist, and tails hang out, but this is of little importance – so why nit-pick?

Criticism in the delicate area of toileting should be avoided whenever possible. It is highly embarrassing for an adult to be caught short by an episode of incontinence. Similarly it is a blow to a small person's pride and self-confidence. It is important not to rub it in but to treat the slip-up casually and move on quickly.

Early days at school

Starting school is a strange, exciting time and Jessica came home the first day with uncomfortably wet knickers. Little boys do not cope any better, and accidents are to be expected. Sometimes it is because your small-timer is too shy to put his hand up and ask to be excused. He may be afraid about using a strange toilet.

Jessica
Jessica was always afraid that she would get locked in a strange toilet and find herself unable to undo the catch, so she tried to wait until she got home. Her bladder could not stand up to the increasing pressure and all the urine flooded out. Reassurance was all that she needed – and practice with the tricky catches.

JUNIORS
Bed-wetting

Enuresis, from the Greek, is a formal term for bed-wetting, used for children of school age and older people. It is often called nocturnal enuresis since the likeliest time for control to break down is at night, during sleep, but it can also occur in the day.

Secondary enuresis comes on after a period when the child had been dry. A common and obvious cause is a urinary infection such as cystitis. The urine is cloudy and passing it stings or burns, but the disorder is usually quickly dealt with by a few days on an antibiotic. Other physical illnesses, especially those involving a fever, can also cause secondary bed-wetting, but in most cases the cause is emotional, with insecurity a key factor.

Lucy
Lucy's insecurity sprang from starting at a big, new school after the cosy little nursery school – and her special friend was going to a different school.

Philip
Philip was upset by his parents' break-up. He missed seeing his father, refused to eat his supper and rebelled against going to bed. He woke up wet with tears and wet with urine.

Janie
Janie felt threatened by the arrival of the new baby who was already claiming a lot of her mother's time. It looked as though there was a high risk of a take-over. Her reaction was to regress to baby ways – crawling, dribbling and wetting and asking for a bottle.

Peter
Peter had been very fond of his grandmother and when she died he slipped back into wetting himself, and like Janie he would not eat food that he normally enjoyed. Gran had made gingerbread men and other small treats, but more importantly, she was a major part of his support system.

The reassuring aspect of secondary enuresis is that the child has previously been dry, so you know that it is not a physical impossibility.

The cure – the essential ingredients are love and limitless patience, optimism about the outcome and a generally calm, matter-of-fact attitude. Impatience is counter-productive and prolongs the process and there is no place for discipline in relation to bladder and bowel control.

Very late primary enuresis occurs in a few unhappy children, often those who have been ill or disturbed at the critical time for acquiring control. They will nearly always get the hang of it in the end with no special treatment but time. There is a second burst of maturing in the genitourinary area – sex and water – at around 11, the beginning of puberty. A child who really wants to be dry may find the pad and buzzer helps. It lets him know when the pad begins to get damp and gradually his body learns to anticipate the buzz. Similarly, we adults often wake up just in time to switch off the alarm clock.

Some children respond to stars stuck on a sheet of paper to record the dry nights, others to an accumulation of points which earn a bigger reward. The emphasis is always on the positive. You don't expect to win the jackpot every time, but each dry night is a step in the right direction and a cause for greater confidence.

Making too much of a fuss over every success is a mistake, however. It is desirable that the youngster should be dry through the night, but it is something you expect your child to take for granted in the end – like everybody else.

Trouble with the motions – soiling

Most little ones learn to control their motions a few weeks earlier than their water. While urine can soak into a soft warm diaper unnoticed, it is difficult for a toddler not to be aware of solid waste in his or her nappy or pants when walking around. This is the trigger for her learning to take charge herself and try using the pot.

The commonest problem with the bowels is constipation, which might seem a far cry from incontinence. The constipated motions are dry and hard and difficult to pass. They may scratch or tear the delicate membrane lining the anus, making a crack called an *anal fissure*. This is acutely painful when the child goes to the loo, so she puts it off . . . and off, making the constipation worse, and the stool even harder. Paradoxically, this in turn can lead to a form of incontinence. Liquid motions, dammed up behind a blockage, escape round the sides, but the sufferer has no control over them.

Only very rarely is anal incontinence due to slow or late development. Constipation can start after a feverish illness in which the body sweats off too much water leaving the colon and the motions dry. Often, however, soiling is the cry for help of a disturbed child – perhaps upset by the arrival of a baby brother or sister, a potential usurper of her position and her mother's time and attention. Moving house, being cared for temporarily by a stranger or even an aunty, are other upsetting events. Soiling is often partly a reaction to an over-enthusiastic potty training regime.

To deal with soiling, whatever its origins, the first essential is to accept the messy youngster affectionately, with no hint of disgust, to foster a sense of security and trust between adult and child. The backdrop needs to be easy-going.

Urging the youngster to try harder to pass a motion in the right place does not work, but a teaspoonful of Milk of Magnesia may help by softening the motion and also psychologically. Beating a soiling problem takes as long as it takes. The vital thing is for the youngster to feel well loved.

Constipation itself needs addressing. A faulty diet contributes to it. Such popular foods as sweets, chocolate, crisps, ice-cream, biscuits and cake are all highly palatable and easy to eat. They provide nourishment but too little fibre for the colon to get a grip on. Vegetables, fruit and bran, plus plenty of water, give the bowel what it needs.

Stanley
Stanley had a wretched time at school. As a soiler, he was the butt of hurtful comments. No one wanted to sit next to him because he smelled. When he was two and had just learned some bowel and bladder control, his mother died. Stanley was shunted from relative to relative, then to a series of foster homes, an angry, despairing little boy. Partly from defiance, partly involuntarily, he often emptied his bowels at the wrong time, in the wrong place. This went on. The breakthrough came when he was changing and

JUNIORS

developing physically and coincidentally came under the care of a sympathetic teacher who had had similar but milder problems as a child.

Toilet training

This means helping your child out of the incontinence of the very young, something your child will largely do for herself at the right stage in her personal development. All you have to do is provide the right equipment and a warm, mildly encouraging atmosphere – when she is ready.

Guidelines
- Do not make the mistake of potting your baby as early as possible, but wait until she gives the signal that she is aware that puddles are somehow to do with her. She will be an established walker, and probably 20–22 months old – although the 'right' age is an individual matter.
- Do not start training when there is a major event happening – such as a new baby or a new house.
- Dish out praise in a casual manner and give no signs of disappointment at failures. Overdoing your concern either way puts extra pressure on the learner, leading to tension and loss of control.
- Never show disgust.

Toileting timetable for the learner

Plan regular, sufficiently frequent opportunities to use the pot without hurry or hassle. The big loo with a seat on top often suits best. A reasonable programme is three times a day after meals, shortly before bedtime and whenever your little one asks. It is also worthwhile to lift her when you go to bed. Probably she won't wake up but will pass water as a reflex when she feels the cold pot touching her bottom.

If the training does not go smoothly, and 'accidents' keep occurring, keep your cool and go into a reduced expectation mode. A physical illness can be expected to put back the programme, and also check for emotional stress – for instance the death of a pet.

6
Adolescents

Adolescents are agonizingly sensitive. They are acutely aware of their bodies which are going through amazing changes in size and shape and powers. The flood of sex hormones reaches its peak. For boys there are their new, unpredictable, croaking voices; for girls there is the monthly bleed triggered by the release of an ovum and with the practical possibility of becoming pregnant.

Until this twenty-first-century generation of youngsters, 13 and 14 year olds were still children. Today a 13 year old, or even an 11 or 12 year old, will be sexually aware, while a significant minority have experience of intercourse. At 15 most young people of both sexes are no longer innocents. This subjects them to enormous strains. We hear of boys who have become fathers at 12, and girls, in record numbers in the UK, only too frequently becoming pregnant while they are still at school. To add to the tension, these are also the years of important examinations.

Teenagers today are well versed in the physical facts of sexual relations but may be overwhelmed emotionally. They get little guidance from their elders, who in turn have lost the rigid moral framework of their parents and grandparents. The stresses the young are subjected to make them anxious to conform precisely with the standards of their peers. They fret endlessly about any perceived deviation from the norm – in their personal appearance, clothes, and interests. They are desperate to be like everybody else, including the function of their bodies. No way can it be considered cool to be incontinent.

It causes great distress at 70, but unimaginable humiliation for a girl or boy of 17. Sadly, it happens quite frequently. Tough, healthy, sporty youngsters are no more immune than the wimps and the weaklings, but most vulnerable are those who were slow to acquire all-night dryness as small-timers.

Charlie
Charlie (for Charlotte) was a leading light on the tennis court at 15. The first time she found her pants were wet after a match, she

put it down to the excitement of the game, a once-off. But it wasn't an isolated incident. It happened increasingly often and it became a matter of anxiety in case she left a tell-tale damp patch when she was sitting with the others, after the game.

It wasn't only active sport that caused a leakage. A bout of coughing could do it, and on one shameful occasion she was helping her form mistress to move a table when she felt a horrible warm trickle down her inner thigh. Charlie's trouble was stress incontinence, the type brought on by increased pressure in the abdomen, automatically raising the pressure in the bladder. This usually comes from tensing the abdominal muscles, either on purpose or by coughing, sneezing or laughing. Stress incontinence can occur at any age but when the leaking only happens with laughter it may have a totally different cause.

Giggle incontinence

Giggle incontinence, or to give it its scientific name, *enuresis risoria*, is not uncommon, but it only affects teenage girls, and is always set off by laughing. Although this odd disorder has long been recognized, why it happens remains something of a mystery. Raised pressure in the bladder is not involved. Instead there is a sudden relaxation of the urethral sphincter, as though the power had been switched off, allowing the urine in the bladder to escape. There is nothing the girl can do to stop it until the giggling settles down.

The favourite theory suggests that the fault lies in the nervous system, not in the plumbing. Something similar can happen in older people after a stroke. In both cases the nerves simply stop carrying the appropriate messages to the muscles responsible for closing off the bladder.

It is important to distinguish between ordinary stress incontinence and the giggle variety, because effective management differs in each type. In the stress kind there is a range of circumstances that can lead to leakage, especially physical exercise. The fault is weakness of the sphincter and the muscles of the pelvic floor. Treatment is directed at strengthening the latter by specific exercises and re-education of the bladder so that it tolerates increasingly long periods between visits to the loo (see pp. 7–8).

ADOLESCENTS

Estelle

Estelle, aged 16, was disconcerted to find that whenever her friend Barbara came round she could not control her water. They often laughed 'until they cried' at the same jokes, but neither Estelle nor her doctor realized at first that it was the fits of the giggles that also made her lose control of her bladder.

The good news is that girls always grow out of enuresis risoria. Women over 25-plus never develop it. However, strong emotion can affect the bladder at any age.

Bladder instability – dyssynergia

Although stress incontinence and the adolescent 'giggle' type are the most likely to affect the 12–20 age group, some girls and a few boys develop urge incontinence. They cannot wait. The cause is an unstable bladder, particularly affecting the detrusor (emptying) muscle in the bladder wall. It fails to respond appropriately to the pressure inside the bladder as it fills. Instead it contracts spasmodically at any stage during the filling, often without the usual advance warning sensation, and there is an urgent need to pass water. Bladder instability often first shows itself as a long-term problem in teens.

Unduly rapid filling of the bladder due to water tablets (diuretics), alcohol or too much fluid may precipitate urge incontinence, as may irritation of the bladder by a stone or inflammation. Cutting down on excess fluid, especially tea, coffee and alcohol, is a sensible precaution. Specific treatment is described on p. 85. Fortunately, when the sexual organs develop during puberty, the adjacent parts of the urinary system also increase in size and maturity. Retraining of the bladder stands a good chance of success at this stage, even in apparently intractable enuresis.

Psychological stress

The years from the turmoil of puberty, that is growing up physically and becoming established as an adult at 20-plus, are notorious for intense emotions and sensitivity. Thoughts and feelings rebound on the urinary system. We have all had the experience of wanting to pass water more often than usual before an important examination or other ordeal, or when we are physically scared. This normal reaction is seen throughout the mammalian kingdom. For instance, if a stranger walks into a field where there is a flock of sheep their immediate reaction to the potential danger is to urinate.

Adolescents are especially prone to frequency and urgency in a situation of psychological stress. A teenager or an adult who is chronically tense and nervous may develop a hypersensitivity to quite a small amount of urine in the bladder. They may also suffer from *nocturia*, the need to get up and pass water in the night.

Bobby
Bobby had wet his bed until he was six, a little late, and was still a nail-biter at 13. He was always asking to go to the loo at the most inconvenient times. When his parents' marriage was going through a rough patch Bobby's frequency got worse and the night they had a row he wet his bed for the first time for four years. The Child Guidance Clinic helped him and his parents reduce his anxiety and reassure him they were not going to split up.

Coital incontinence

The sexual freedom that exploded in the sixties affected adolescent behaviour more than any other. This has had disadvantages. Because the youngsters can and do have intercourse while they are still emotionally immature they are susceptible to coital incontinence. This is the reaction of passing water involuntarily during the act, an embarrassing reminder to empty the bladder before sex. The trigger to the incontinence is the moment of entry of the penis, against a backdrop of a high state of excitement. Experience and maturity are the best preventives.

7
Seniors

A tendency to leak is common among seniors but you don't have to accept it as inevitable or untreatable. All through our lives our bodies and minds are changing and adjusting the better to suit our needs. Growth and development dominate the first 25 years, followed by another 25 years of consolidation at first of our physical powers but increasingly of intellectual interests and knowledge. The third and fourth ages are the senior years.

The gradual changes that characterize this period are geared to smooth and economical running, cutting out non-essentials and redundancies, and living with the minimum expenditure of energy, as befits a pensioner. Seventy year olds and older do not want all the paraphernalia of child care, so they do not need such a big supply of the hormones that previously kept the reproductive system ready for action. The most important of these hormones is oestrogen, which has effects all over the body.

The skin

Nowhere are the changes of ageing clearer than in the skin. It becomes thinner, from a reduction in the amount of collagen, a protein supporting the skin and other tissues, giving them solidity, strength and lubrication. Older skin is drier and more delicate than before. You don't see seniors with spotty, greasy or sweaty complexions.

Fining down is a general effect of ageing all over the body. The hair becomes less abundant, the pubic hair practically disappears, and the individual hairs become finer. An economy in brown, black or red pigment leaves the hair grey or white, and the skin, too, becomes paler. You rarely see a tanned face and body in an 80 year old, but fair-skinned people tend to develop large, irregular freckles on their hands and forearms.

SENIORS

Phyllis

Phyllis was running a one-woman campaign against age. She watched her diet, religiously eating the five fruits a day and restricting all sweet and fatty foods and took the recommended 40-minute walk three times a week. She exercised her brain with the crossword in her daily paper. It did not seem fair that when she was only 60 the incontestable signs of ageing began to appear – where they were most noticeable, in her hair and skin.

Her dark hair was touched with snow, and her face had become paler, but it was the wrinkles round her eyes that bothered her and the definite sag, blurring her jaw line. Hair dye made her look like a witch, and thicker cosmetics only emphasized the changes in her skin. Phyllis accepted all this, but the episodes of incontinence made her feel ashamed and afraid to go out.

The determination she called into play to persevere with her diet and the walks, she now transferred to the pelvic floor exercises which the incontinence nurse taught her. Over a period of six months she regained a useful degree of control, and kept it with continuing exercises.

The bladder

Some hollow organs, like the womb and the bladder, undergo a general decrease in size akin to the thinning of the skin. The shrinkage of the womb is irrelevant at this age but the reduced capacity of the bladder can be inconvenient. It fills more rapidly which means going to the loo more often – frequency – and an increased risk of overflow incontinence. The likelihood of developing cystitis – inflammation of the bladder – increases with age, especially in women, with their short run between the bladder and the outside. It is usually caused by an infection travelling up the urethra and is a major cause of urge incontinence, by irritating the bladder.

The vagina

The lining of the vagina shares with the skin its increasing dryness and delicacy, which is even more marked because it is thin and fragile to start with. This is known as *vaginal atrophy* and frequently develops into *vaginitis* or inflammation. Unlike cystitis it is not due to an infection, but to a shortage of oestrogen now the ovaries have retired. The vagina is particularly susceptible to this lack and becomes dry, red and sore, making intercourse painful – even with lashings of KY jelly or other lubrication. The all-over shrinkage in size makes matters even more uncomfortable and the irritation by the more concentrated urine is a further trigger to urge incontinence. Some people make matters worse by cutting down on the amount they drink, concentrating the urine even more.

Nocturia is another result of shrinkage and irritation. It means having to get up to pass water in the night. More urine is produced at night than in the day, averaging 400 ml. While for a man getting up once in the night is the normal maximum, it is twice for a woman.

Fortunately help is at hand in the form of several locally effective preparations of oestrogen. There are creams and ointments to apply such as dienoestrol and ring-pessaries; and vaginal tablets containing oestrogen. They provide considerable relief and do not affect other parts of the body, such as the uterus. Plants known as phyto-oestrogens, especially soya beans, supply small amounts of the hormone if taken by mouth and this may be enough to make up for the shortfall.

Producing less oestrogen is part of the body's economy drive. While seniors do not need to keep the baby production line in working order, they may well enjoy an extended active sex life now that we all live so much longer. The strengthening effect of oestrogen on the vaginal lining is required as much as ever.

Sometimes, as a precursor to the dryness of vaginitis, there may be a watery pink discharge which may be mistaken for incontinence.

Maturity-onset diabetes

This disorder has become almost epidemic in recent years with an ageing population. Since the main symptoms are thirst, leading to drinking a lot, causing in turn frequency of micturition (passing water), any tendency to incontinence is made worse. Often it is the first clue to the diagnosis of diabetes, a disease in which there is too much sugar in the blood. Treatment involves controlling this by diet and by drugs known as hypoglycaemics which reduce the blood glucose (sugar) level. Examples are glibenclamide and metformin. Insulin injections are needed in severe cases. Everyone with diabetes needs to take meticulous care to avoid infections, especially of the skin. The bugs thrive on the sweetness.

A serious effect of diabetes on the urinary system is damage to the nerves that control the bladder, leading to instability of the detrusor muscle. This is a potent cause of urge incontinence. Difficulty in emptying the bladder may be another result of nerve damage and paradoxically this can also lead to incontinence, but of the overflow type.

Arthritis and osteoporosis

These common, progressive, crippling conditions of the later years can have an indirect effect on urinary continence – holding one's water. When movement is slow and painful there is anxiety about getting to the toilet in time. This enhances the sense of urgency and increases the risk of incontinence. The worst time is often first thing when there is maximum stiffness of the joints and the muscles including the detrusor. Added to that is the effect of gravity on changing from the horizontal to the vertical position (see pp. 2, 45). A bedside commode or a bottle, adapted for either sex, can save a lot of wet beds.

Muscle weakness

The gradual loss of muscle cells and their replacement with inelastic fibres causes increasing muscular weakness from around the early fifties. This adds to the crippling effects of arthritis and also involves the detrusor muscle. The weaker contractions of the bladder mean that it takes longer to empty and visits to the toilet are more frequent. The likelihood of infection getting in is enhanced.

Constipation

Sluggish bowels are one of the common problems of older people, and weakness of the abdominal muscles is a contributory factor. A diet that depends on refined carbohydrates – cakes, buns and biscuits with sugar on everything – is often adopted by elderly women living alone. It saves the trouble of cooking and requires very little chewing, a plus point for those with poor teeth; but it unbalances the diet and does nothing to keep the colon healthily active. Salads, fruit and vegetables, bran and wholegrain cereals such as oats are not popular with most seniors, but they contain the fibre that provides the bulk that stimulates the bowel. Meat dishes are also stimulating.

The rule of five, advocated by the Government, recommends eating five portions of vegetables and fruit every day. It is an excellent recipe for combating constipation. General exercise, for instance half-an-hour's walk daily, brisk if possible, also helps. Constipation can lead to stress incontinence when straining is involved. It can also lead to overflow incontinence if hard lumps of waste matter in the rectum press on the urethra and block the outflow of urine.

Adverse effects of smoking, drinking and some medication on the risk of incontinence

- *Smoking* irritates the bladder and can make an unstable bladder worse.
- *Alcohol* has a double effect – stimulating the kidneys to make more urine and the bladder to pass water more often – frequency and incontinence. Beer is worse than wines and spirits because of the greater volume.
- *Caffeine* is the essential stimulant in coffee, tea (containing only half as much), cola and other fizzy drinks, while cocoa contains a similar chemical. Their diuretic effect can lead to incontinence.
- *Citrus drinks* stimulate the bladder, also leading to an increased chance of urge incontinence.

Drugs affecting bladder control

- *Diuretics* are intended to step up the volume of urine passed so as to relieve excess fluid throwing a burden on the body, for instance in high blood pressure, kidney failure, heart failure and swollen ankles, from less serious causes. Some, such as spironolactone (Aldactide), have a short, sharp effect useful in urgent situations, while others, for example triamterene (Dyazide) or bendrofluazide (Aprinox) are milder. Sometimes they work too well, resulting in frequency, urgency and leakage.

- *Sleepers, pain-killers and some antidepressants* such as clomipramine (Anafranil) and anxiolytics such as lorazepam (Ativan) or diazepam (Valium) dull down bodily sensations so that the information that the bladder is full may not get through to consciousness. A wet bed may result. Medicines used to damp down the cough centre, antitussives, may have the same effect. Spinal and epidural injections, given as anaesthesia during surgery, may lead to temporary incontinence afterwards.

Some medicines are given specifically to prevent the person sleeping too deeply to wake when the bladder fills. They include anticholinergic drugs, for instance oxybutynin (Cystrin) and some antidepressants, especially imipramine (Tofranil), which relax the bladder and reduce the frequency of needing to pass water. Antispasmodics such as flavoxate (Urispas) have a similar effect. Desmopressin, given as a nasal spray or in tablet form, acts on the control of nocturia by mimicking the hormone that has been shown to be lacking in some sufferers.

The problem with the drugs aimed at preventing incontinence is that they may cause retention – that is, you cannot pass water although you have the urge. It can be sudden and painful, requiring prompt relief with a catheter, or milder and longer term. In this case the bladder remains full but overflows. If this goes on continuously it is called 'dribble incontinence'. Treatment starts with catheterization, followed by investigation of the cause.

Tumours

Tumours – lumps or swellings inside the bladder – can cause irritation and urge incontinence. They may be harmless polyps or cancerous growths, which are most likely to occur in the age span 60–70. Bladder cancer is three times as common in men as in women, and is the fourth commonest male cancer. Together with cancer of the prostate it accounts for nearly all cancers of the urinary system.

Smoking increases the risk fourfold and contributes to a third of the cases while another third are caused by industrial chemicals. Chronic cystitis or bladder stones also increase the risk. The key symptom, one that should alert you, is blood in the urine, *haematuria*. The diagnosis is confirmed by an ultrasound picture of the bladder or a *urogram*, an X-ray of the water system when it is filled with a fluid that shows up.

The treatment is resection – surgery to remove the tumour, or destroying it with diathermy, burning by an electric current.

8
Special problems – prolapse, fistula and fibroids

Prolapse

Prolapse means slipping down from the normal position and usually refers to the pelvic organs. With our upright posture, the force of gravity puts a constant strain on the pelvic floor. This mix of strips of muscle, ligaments and fibres – all soft tissues – has to support the womb and the other contents of the pelvis. Sometimes it gives way to a greater or lesser extent – prolapse. There are several types and degrees. The organs that may be involved are the bladder, the urethra, the uterus, the rectum and, most importantly, the vagina.

A *cystocoele* occurs when the upper two-thirds of the front wall of the vagina gives way and brings part of the bladder down with it. If the lower third is involved it is a *urethrocoele*. A *rectocoele* is the bulging forward of the rectum into the back of the vagina. A *rectal prolapse* is something quite different; it does not involve the vagina and consists of part of the lining of the rectum poking out of the back passage. *Uterine prolapse* means that the uterus has slipped down into the vagina. There are three degrees:

1 The womb and cervix move only a short way down the vagina.
2 The cervix protrudes from the vagina.
3 The whole womb has come out through the vagina. Third degree prolapse is also known as *procidentia*, Latin for falling down forwards.

Prolapse of whichever type or degree is much likelier if you have had children, especially several. It usually presents itself during the perimenopause, the menopause, or the postmenopausal stage, which extends indefinitely.

Symptoms

Incontinence is frequently the key symptom but it is occasionally possible to have prolapse without incontinence or vice versa. The next commonest effect is the feeling of 'something coming down', a

SPECIAL PROBLEMS – PROLAPSE, FISTULA AND FIBROIDS

definite lump between the legs, or merely an uneasy, physically insecure feeling that is difficult to pinpoint.

Causes

- *Damage* to the pelvic ligaments which normally anchor the uterus in place. A long or difficult labour involves excessive stretching of these ligaments, so that they lose their elasticity. Generally, however, they recover within three months of the birth.
- *Lack of oestrogen* because of the menopause leaves the tissues weaker, so that they recover less well.
- *Raised pressure inside the abdomen* stresses the supports of the uterus and vagina and throws a strain on the mechanism for preventing leakage of urine. In this situation the sudden extra pressure of laughing or coughing may be enough to allow some urine to leak. Long-term causes of raised pressure include obesity, a chronic cough or frequent straining due to constipation. Prolapse is less of a problem in countries where you squat to pass a motion.

Prolapse is not painful but unpleasantly uncomfortable and often accompanied by backache. The symptoms are worse during the day, when you are standing up and gravity operates. Lying down to rest is a relief, but sexual intercourse may be excruciating. Neither pain nor bleeding from the vagina result from prolapse and if they occur in the course of the disorder a full investigation is needed to find the cause.

Diagnosis

This depends on the symptoms and vaginal examination. Traditionally the latter is carried out with the patient lying on her left side. She is asked to cough, which shows up stress incontinence at once, and the doctor can feel the position of the womb with two fingers in the vagina.

Treatment

Prophylaxis, or prevention, calls for:

- careful stitching of tears during labour
- regular pelvic floor exercises (see pp. 54, 55, 84–5)
- correction of constipation, and overhaul of the diet accordingly
- reduction of excess weight

SPECIAL PROBLEMS – PROLAPSE, FISTULA AND FIBROIDS

- not smoking

Ongoing treatment can be:

- hormone replacement therapy (HRT), especially if there are symptoms of oestrogen lack
- local oestrogen treatment with pessaries (silicone rings) or vaginal tablets
- surgery (see p. 77)

Margery
Margery was 43 when she first noticed a feeling like a lump in her vagina. It did not hurt but it seemed to get in the way when she was passing a motion, and she felt a similar obstruction when she had intercourse. This was particularly upsetting because, although she had two lovely daughters, she wanted to have one more try for a boy. Her family doctor referred her to a gynaecologist who asked her about problems with the births of her children, episodes of incontinence, how often she passed a motion, any attacks of cystitis and what medicines she was taking (none). He also tested her urine, but it was the vaginal examination that clinched the diagnosis.

Margery had a uterine prolapse, stage 1, with the complication of urge incontinence. The doctor explained the treatment options, having found that she enjoyed an active sexual life and wanted it to be possible to have another child. Although a hysterectomy would certainly cure the prolapse it would finish any chance of pregnancy. She tried for three months using a ring pessary in the hope of it supporting the uterus. This is sometimes enough with a slight prolapse but not in Margery's case.

The treatment she chose was a repair of the over-stretched vagina and a repositioning of the bladder and urethra which had also slipped out of place. She turned out to be one of the 60 per cent in whom such operations are successful in the relief of incontinence as well as correcting the prolapse.

Fistula

A fistula – Latin for a pipe – is an abnormal passageway between two organs or with the outside world. It can occur as an error of development and is then called congenital since the baby is born with it. It can also be produced by the erosion of a sore or weak place in the organs concerned; but in Western civilization a fistula is usually the result of radiotherapy for cancer or a direct effect of the cancer itself. Sometimes accidental damage during a hysterectomy causes a fistula. A bright spot is that fistulae may heal spontaneously.

Vesicovaginal fistula is a rare connection between the bladder and the vagina. It allows urine to travel from the bladder into the vagina, by-passing the anti-leak arrangement of the urethral sphincter. The result is continuous incontinence. The only effective treatment is surgical repair approached either through the vagina or by an incision in the abdomen.

Colovesical fistula links the bowel (colon) and bladder and causes continuous incontinence through the back passage. It is also liable to cause infection of the bladder with gut bacteria – cystitis. Antibiotics are needed before a surgical repair can be carried out.

Fibroids

A fibroid is a very common non-cancerous growth or tumour of the muscular wall of the uterus. It can occur singly or there may be several. Harmless in itself, it may cause symptoms by pressing on the surrounding tissues. A large fibroid may squash the urethra, occasionally causing retention of urine and overflow incontinence. Urgency, frequency and urge incontinence may also result from the pressure of a fibroid. Other possible symptoms include painful periods and an extra loss of blood.

Fluid in the vagina from vaginitis is an uncommon symptom ometimes accompanying a fibroid (see pp. 18, 39–40).

Treatment

The two main reasons for having a hysterectomy are heavy bleeding from the uterus without an obvious cause and fibroids. Fibroids themselves often lead to excessive bleeding because they increase the surface area of the lining of the uterus. The one certain cure for fibroids is a hysterectomy, but apart from frequent psychological problems, there is the irrevocable end to having babies. There are no medical treatments that dispose of fibroids, but a lesser operation to remove only the fibroid or fibroids can often be successful. This is a *myomectomy* from the Greek, *my* means muscle, *oma* tumour and *ektome* cutting out.

Sue

Sue's major problem was flooding, but she also had painful periods. She was only 41 and was horrified to develop urge incontinence. With an internal examination, the doctor found that her uterus was extra bulky and diagnosed fibroids, probably several. Sue said she would feel only half a woman if she had her womb removed so she chose to have a myomectomy. Her symptoms improved and she had less blood loss, but her periods were still painful. She welcomed the change.

Multiple sclerosis

Multiple sclerosis is one of the commonest diseases of the brain and nervous system. It comprises a scattering, throughout the system, of patches of scar-like tissue which interrupt the messages travelling down the nerves. This makes for a variety of symptoms of which some of the most troublesome are those affecting the bladder.

The controls no longer work properly and the bladder fails in both of its functions – storing urine securely until it gets the go-ahead to pass it, and emptying itself effectively and completely. One likely result is that urine leaks out almost continuously or in spontaneous episodes as the bladder fills partway. Frequency and urgency – you can't wait – are part of the syndrome. The other reaction is the opposite. You want and need to pass water but cannot get the message through and are left with a full bladder.

With the first alternative, incontinence, several medicines, including oxybutynin, and the usual ploys, such as using pads and not drinking at bedtime, are helpful. It is also good sense to empty your bladder at regular intervals, say every two hours initially (see p. 83). When the problem is difficulty in emptying the bladder completely, the only effective way of managing is by catheter. Self-catheterization is not as difficult as it sounds and you soon get the knack of it. It has the great advantage of restoring your independence.

Because of the random distribution of the patches of sclerosis

SPECIAL PROBLEMS – PROLAPSE, FISTULA AND FIBROIDS

interrupting the nerves there is no regular group of symptoms in MS, but typically there may be *dysarthria*, difficulty in speaking, *ataxia*, unsteadiness in walking and other movements, and *nystagmus*, flicking of the eyes to one side. Signs that make it likely that any symptoms are due to MS include tingling in the spine and limbs when you bend your neck forwards, and worsening of the symptoms after exercise or when you have a temperature.

Jeremy
Jeremy was 42. His first attack of MS had been 12 years before, and like most first attacks affected his eyes among other symptoms. It lasted three months. Since then he has alternated between attacks and periods of remission when the problems vanish and he seems perfectly normal. Remission can last a matter of weeks or go on for years. Currently, Jeremy has been well for four years – a record for him. Treatment with numerous drugs seems to improve matters for a while, including the urinary difficulties, but there is no cure.

Stroke

A stroke, or *cardiovascular attack* (CVA), is another common disorder affecting the brain, including the water control system. Unlike MS, it is easy to identify, the symptoms usually coming on over a few minutes and reaching the maximum disability in 1–2 hours. The cause is either the blockage of a major artery or serious bleeding from it, usually associated with high blood pressure. The result is *hemiparesis* – weakness or paralysis on one side of the body, more often the left. There may be problems with speech and finding the right word among a variety of other possible symptoms.

Incontinence frequently accompanies the early phases of a stroke, but does not necessarily persist. Some practical problems may compound the difficulties with bladder control – for instance impaired mobility because of weakness so that you cannot hurry to the loo. You may also have lost your manual dexterity on one side so that you cannot manage your clothes, using toilet paper, or a bottle. Speech problems and problems with comprehension can interfere with your communicating with other people – including telling them your needs regarding toileting.

SPECIAL PROBLEMS – PROLAPSE, FISTULA AND FIBROIDS

Time is on your side after a stroke. All the symptoms tend to improve steadily for as long as a year, but it requires continuous effort on your part and all the help you can get. Most valuable are physiotherapists and speech therapists combined with an incontinence adviser, usually a nurse, to teach you the pelvic floor exercises, bladder drill and some other tricks for improving control.

9
Pregnancy and childbirth

Incontinence from time to time is a common reaction in the first three months of pregnancy and again in the last month and for up to three months after the birth. In many women childbirth triggers a chronic tendency to leakiness – unless positive action is taken.

Early in pregnancy, in fact within seven days of conception, even before you have missed a period, the kidneys start making more urine than usual. This is in response to hormonal signals about the exciting new developments in the womb. They set off a whole train of events, starting with increased frequency. This is not only due to the extra water but also to the irritating effect of the enlarging uterus crowding the bladder. The pregnancy hormone, progesterone, kicks in, calming your mood and relaxing the soft tissues in the bony pelvis. These are the muscles and ligaments that support the uterus and hold it in position. The joints between the bones of the pelvis, which usually have very little movement, become more flexible in readiness for the birth.

Among the muscles that are relaxed is the urethral sphincter, which keeps the bladder watertight in the ordinary way. Now it is more liable to leak with any extra pressure. As the uterus enlarges it presses on the bladder, leading to stress incontinence, the type in which urine escapes when you cough or laugh. Frequency and urgency often occur too, and urge incontinence may develop.

The all-round pressure on the bladder in the tight confines of the pelvis can make it more difficult to empty the bladder completely – partial urinary retention. This enhances the risk of an infection taking hold and causing cystitis in early pregnancy. From around the twelfth week morning sickness peters out, ushering in the most comfortable period of pregnancy. The uterus rises out of the bony pelvic cage and the pressure on the bladder is relieved. Incontinence is less of a nuisance during the next 2–3 months. However, one in every three women is incontinent at some time in her reproductive years, and an embarrassing leakage is common in the weeks running up to labour. It normally stops with the birth of the baby, but in over a third of new mothers it continues for as long as three months afterwards.

PREGNANCY AND CHILDBIRTH

Anne

Anne was 30. She and John had been live-in partners for nearly two years and for the last six months they had been trying for a baby. Anne had stopped taking the Pill and was disappointed when nothing happened. Her doctor said it sometimes takes several cycles after giving up the contraceptive before the hormones recover their rhythm. She tried not to be too optimistic – until her period was three weeks overdue.

The first symptoms she noticed were waves of nausea, not only in the mornings, and a tender, pricking feeling in her breasts. They felt heavy. She felt tired, even exhausted, at any time of day, and occasionally faint or dizzy. Oddities were a metallic taste in her mouth, and the way she went right off coffee and developed a passion for cucumber sandwiches.

The pregnancy test from the chemist confirmed what she already suspected from her symptoms. Around the twelfth week Anne became aware that she was running to the loo more often than usual, but this became less frequent over the next month or two. Later, as the expected date of delivery (EDD) drew near, the foetus grew fast and Anne's abdomen became larger. She began to have episodes of leakage as the womb crowded her bladder and her trips to the loo were more frequent again. After some hours of fruitless labour, the baby was born with the help of forceps.

Often any problems with frequency or incontinence stop at this stage, but Anne was among the 30–40 per cent of mothers who are troubled with leaks for 2–3 months after giving birth. Her urethral sphincter and the muscles of the pelvic floor had all been weakened by the long labour and she was a candidate for stress incontinence. Guided by the maternity nurse Anne started on a programme of pelvic floor exercises. She will have to keep them up for many months, probably indefinitely, to keep the problem under control. Ideally, she would have started them during the pregnancy but it is never too late to benefit.

Pregnancy and childbirth throw a huge stretching strain on the tissues surrounding the baby, weakening the muscles and ligaments of the pelvic floor and those of the bladder. These include the structures that support the neck of the bladder and the urethra, parts that are particularly important for maintaining continence. The birth itself can cause tearing of the tissues. Nearly 50 per cent of mothers suffer episodes of incontinence in their middle years.

Stress incontinence, the commonest type, is more likely after a long or difficult labour or a forceps delivery. Even a Caesarian section, which should in theory avoid stress on the mother's tissues, can clock up some damage, especially if it is a second or third such operation. In some cases, if the baby has travelled down the birth canal too fast or with difficulty, the nerves that control the muscles of the pelvic floor are injured. The *pudendal nerve* is the most important. The normal messages carried by these nerves may fail to get through, and automatic emptying of the bladder when it gets full takes over, regardless of the time and convenience.

Urinary retention – inability to empty the bladder – sometimes comes on immediately following a birth, especially if an epidural or spinal injection has been used for the anaesthetic. Such injections produce a loss of sensation including, of course, pain, in the lower part of the body. The effect lasts for 3–5 hours, but the mother remains mentally aware. With no sensation below the waist until the anaesthetic stops working, she has no control over her water – temporarily. Epidurals are increasingly popular among women who want to know and experience first-hand the marvel of birth. They are also given to mothers who would be at increased risk from a general anaesthetic because of a heart or lung disorder. One disadvantage is a slightly increased risk of damage to the pelvic floor, because you cannot feel any pain from straining and tearing.

There is no quick and easy cure for incontinence, or even a surefire preventive. It is a matter of investing time and effort, and most of us don't bother until we have troublesome symptoms. However, if you are pregnant or even contemplating it, get down to preparing your body for the extra demands that will be made on it. The essential is to toughen up the pelvic floor which takes the brunt of the strain, by special exercises. The earlier you begin them the better. Some gynaecologists advise that all girls should learn them at puberty.

For starters it makes good sense to keep your body generally fit and active, for instance by taking regular exercise. A brisk 30–40-minute walk on alternate days, or swimming 2–3 times a week, are excellent for toning up. Some pools run classes especially for pregnant and postnatal women. Care with the diet is also a basic must – making sure of a wide mix of foods without overdoing fatty and sugary dishes.

Pelvic floor exercises

These are the key element in preventing or modifying the development of incontinence or regaining control if you have lost it. In 1948 Dr Arnold Kegel of the University of California in Los Angeles bestowed an invaluable tool on the millions of women with current or potential water problems. He worked out a system of exercises to strengthen the delicate but invisible muscles of the pelvic floor, enabling them to do their job as effectively as possible. Strong muscles are the best defence against overstretching and the consequent liability to incontinence.

Do not expect an instant miracle when you start doing the exercises. It is a matter of a daily slog at them for several months and continuing after that with a maintenance regime – indefinitely. You may not notice any benefit for the first month, but take heart. The exercises have proved successful in women of all ages from teenagers to 80 year olds.

10
Checking out what's wrong

You need treatment if you are losing control of your water and it is becoming a nuisance and an embarrassment. The first step is to make an appointment with your doctor. Do not worry that she will think less of you when you explain why you have come. At least half her elderly patients, and indeed any woman over 40, may have the same trouble, although you won't hear them talk about it. You do not have to struggle alone.

Your help team may include:

- family doctor
- practice nurse
- continence adviser
- district nurse (home visits)
- health visitor (children)
- midwife (pregnancy)
- physiotherapist (exercises and massage)
- occupational therapist (to assess disability – from the incontinence)
- specialists:
  - urologist (waterworks)
  - gynaecologist (women's disorders)
  - geriatrician (age-related problems)

After 'taking the history', medical speak for asking you about yourself and your symptoms, the doctor will give you a physical examination. This will be general, covering heart, lungs, abdomen and joints, plus a special pelvic examination to check for such abnormalities as a prolapse and to test the strength of the pelvic floor. If your symptoms suggest it you will have a neurological examination to find out if the nerves are conveying messages efficiently from your brain to the bladder.

CHECKING OUT WHAT'S WRONG
Analysis of your urine

The specimen is collected midstream preferably, and checked for protein, sugar and acidity, and how concentrated it is. This is quickly done by a dip-stick test which comprises dipping a wooden spatula impregnated with chemicals into the urine sample. It changes colour in the presence of sugar or protein. Examining the urine under the microscope for bacteria shows up an infection. If this is positive it is followed by *culturing*, that is allowing the bacteria to grow on a special jelly and checking which antibiotics kill that particular strain of bug.

Five-day diary or frequency/volume chart

Each day for five days you measure all the liquid you drink, how often you go to the loo to pass water, and how much you pass over 24 hours. Record the results.

In the following case studies all individuals complained of incontinence.

Tina

Tina, who was 50 and rather fat, was found to be drinking more than usual because she was always thirsty – and there was sugar in her water. This all spelled diabetes, and the fact that her mother was diabetic confirmed the diagnosis.

Lorna

Lorna, aged 65, went in constant fear of 'an accident'. She had four grown-up children and had been through a difficult time with the last birth. This weakened her pelvic floor muscles and those of the neck of the bladder – both important for preventing leakage. She began having stress incontinence during the menopausal years and it was getting steadily worse. To reduce the likelihood of leaks, as she hoped, Lorna cut down on the amount of fluid she drank. Her last drink of the day was strictly at 4 p.m. Then she began to develop urge incontinence.

The five-day test showed that her urine was unduly concentrated – and irritating to her bladder. It reacted with urgency and frequency. The concentrated urine also made her bladder more susceptible to infection in the form of cystitis, because it was not properly washed out with so little liquid.

John

John was 60 when he began having problems with his prostate. It had become slower and more difficult to empty his bladder and often some stagnant urine was left behind. What took him to the doctor was the development of frequency and a burning pain on passing water. Examining a sample of his water under the microscope showed up the germs of cystitis, a diagnosis that was quickly and easily made.

Checking for leakage

It is easy to measure how much water you have passed if you are able to measure it in a vessel, but it is trickier when you are leaking into a pad or worse – your underwear.

The pad test

Weigh a dry pad, wear it for an hour, starting with a full bladder. Test the effect when you do exercises, sit, stand, climb the stairs, and finally wash your hands under running water. Then weigh the pad again to find out how much has been leaked. You can also find out which activities cause the most leakage.

Urodynamics

Urodynamics refers to the standard set of tests for assessing how well your bladder is functioning. They can be uncomfortable and embarrassing, but not painful. Start with a full bladder and urinate into a special toilet in the hospital urology clinic that measures the rate of flow of the urine. A transducer or detector is introduced through the urethra into the bladder, and another into the back passage to measure the pressure in each place. The bladder is then filled with warm saline through a catheter, taking not more than five minutes. The pressure inside the bladder is measured at different stages of filling. The back passage reading provides the background pressure.

When the bladder is full again you go through various actions such as coughing, lifting or jumping to assess their effect on the pressure. Any leakage is noted and recorded, with the pressure at the time. Lastly you empty your bladder into the special toilet, measuring the flow rate at the different pressures. This whole urodynamic process takes 20–25 minutes, but in some clinics the

CHECKING OUT WHAT'S WRONG

bladder is allowed to refill naturally. In this case it takes about four hours.

Videourodynamics
Videourodynamics is basically the urodynamic routine monitored by X-ray. It gives information about the neck of the bladder in relation to leakage during coughing and other activities – stress incontinence. This is particularly useful for assessing the situation in people who have had surgery in the pelvic area or a complicated labour.

Ambulatory urodynamics
This means carrying a portable recorder to detect leakage during the normal filling of the bladder, which usually takes around four hours. You carry on with your ordinary activities during this time, noting them down. When the bladder is full you try out various actions and exercises which might provoke incontinence. This procedure may help to clarify the diagnosis of stress incontinence in particular.

Uroflowmetry
Starting with a full bladder you pass urine through a funnel into the flowmeter. This prints out a tracing of the rate of flow and shows the maximum rate, how quickly this is reached, and the average rate. A test takes about 30 minutes. A slow rate of flow can indicate faulty contractions of the bladder, a stone or other blockage of the urethra.

Cystometry

Cystometry means measuring the pressure inside the bladder at different volumes, when completely full and during emptying. The bladder must be full at the start of the investigation. Pressure detectors are introduced into the bladder and the rectum. Warm saline is passed into the bladder, and the pressures recorded while it fills. When it is full the pressures are recorded again during such physical activities as jumping, stooping, coughing and laughing. Finally the bladder is emptied into a toilet that measures the bladder pressure during urination.

Videocystometry
Videocystometry or videocystometrography is the process monitored by X-ray filming with a contrast medium in the saline. It is the most effective method for distinguishing between stress and urge incontinence or the combination.

CHECKING OUT WHAT'S WRONG

Urethral pressure profilometry

This compares the pressure in the bladder with that in the urethra. It involves inserting a catheter into the urethra and passing saline through it into the bladder. The catheter is then removed and replaced by another containing two sensors, one to measure the pressure in the urethra, the other to measure that in the bladder itself. Unless the urethral pressure is more than that inside the bladder, urine will leak out. The final step is the slow, careful withdrawal of the urethral sensor while pressure readings are taken at intervals.

Sometimes there is a narrow place or stricture due to scarring from an attack of cystitis. Other causes of narrowing are pressure by the prostate in a man or from a fibroid in a woman. A stone may become lodged in the urethra and that can produce a build-up of pressure on the bladder side of the stone and very low pressure, or none, in the part past the stone.

Pauline

Pauline, at 40, was puzzled when her flow of urine became weak and slow. A urethral profile indicated a partial blockage. She had suffered several bouts of cystitis over the last year or two so it seemed likely that tough scar tissue had replaced some of the muscle cells of the bladder and urethra. This was confirmed by a urethral profile. For the last part of the test, the gradual removal of the sensor, Pauline had to lie very still. The feeling was unpleasant, but she felt no pain.

Imaging – having a look

A picture is helpful in finding out what is wrong. Unfortunately a plain X-ray shows up the bones but not the soft tissues concerned in incontinence – the bladder, ureters and kidneys. There are two ways of overcoming the problem.

Intravenous urogram

A chemical that shows up in X-rays is injected into a vein in the arm and is filmed by X-ray as it is picked up by the kidneys and passed down the ureters into the bladder. It helps in pinpointing abnormalities and also shows if the urine is travelling the wrong way – up towards the kidneys from the bladder.

CHECKING OUT WHAT'S WRONG

Ultrasound
An ultrasound scan, based on inaudible echoes that are picked up from the various organs in the body, is useful in detecting abnormalities in the bladder or kidneys. It is also convenient for assessing how much urine is in the bladder. It is completely painless and gives you a picture to take away. The most frequent use for ultrasound is for viewing an unborn baby.

Cystoscopy
An optical instrument on the principle of the telescope can be passed up the urethra to obtain a view of the inside of the bladder. The cystoscope may be rigid or flexible. It gives a view of stones, areas of inflammation or tumours. A biopsy or sample of the lining can be taken through a rigid instrument. An anaesthetic, either local or general, is needed for this. After the use of either type of cystoscope you may feel sore for a few days when you pass urine.

It is important to drink plenty of water for the next 24 hours, and some urologists give an antibiotic as a routine at this stage, as insurance against infection.

Magnetic resonance imaging (MRI)
MRI is a type of brain and body scan based on magnetic force. It is used to check for abnormalities in the brain or spinal cord which might lead to incontinence by preventing the normal nerve messages getting through. The investigation begins with an injection that makes the areas of interest show up. The patient lies on a trolley that passes through the centre of a tunnel made of a huge, powerful magnet and an X-ray machine. The resulting picture shows, to an expert eye, faults in the working of the nervous system. Some people find the process claustrophobic, but there is no physical discomfort.

Electromyogram
In electromyogram (EMG) *myo* means muscle and *electro* conveys that it is a tracing of the electric currents produced in muscle. The muscle of crucial importance in keeping the bladder watertight is the urethral sphincter, the ring of muscle that acts like a drawstring. The muscle currents are picked up through electrodes. These come in two styles:

- A *surface electrode* is introduced into the urethra through a catheter and is in contact with its lining.
- A *needle electrode*, which is more accurate, comprises a fine needle passed through the skin or the vagina into the urethral sphincter.

The electrode is connected to a machine that converts the electrical activity in the muscle into a trace on the screen, and a sound. A further assessment of the strength of the urethral sphincter is sometimes made while passing water. If the sphincter is weak, a common state of affairs, especially after having children, you are especially vulnerable to stress incontinence.

11
Coping – aids and appliances

When you suffer from incontinence you suffer most of all from a social disability. You are hampered from straying too far from a toilet and you are constantly anxious in case your bladder control lets you down in public. The ideal solution is to cure the problem and in many cases this is possible – sometimes by months of exercises, occasionally with medication and in selected cases with an operation.

There is no instant cure, but there is instant help available. This is where aids and appliances come in. They don't banish the incontinence but they make it manageable. You find you can cope with a reasonably full social life.

Vaginal occlusion devices

You may often have wished you could simply put a stopper in your bladder or shut it off through your vagina. Well, you can. Such appliances are available for the younger woman, say 45 or under, who wants to lead an energetic, sporty life. There are two methods.

Vaginal sponge

The urethra or urine pipe can be blocked by a sponge into the vagina. The sponge is moistened then squeezed dry and introduced into the vagina with a special applicator. It is positioned so as to lift the neck of the bladder, through the vaginal wall, and support the sphincter muscle so that it works to the best advantage. Once in the vagina the sponge expands and presses on the urethra, also preventing any leakage. The procedure is as easy as using a tampon, but the sponge should not be left in situ for any longer than is necessary for the game or exercise session to be completed.

Left in for too long the sponge makes the vagina too dry and its delicate lining becomes sore.

Urethral plug

A small silicone stopper is inserted into the opening of the urethra, acting like any other stopper. It is held in place by a tiny balloon which is inflated through a syringe when it is in the bladder. It requires manual dexterity and skill to insert the balloon, and also to remove it. You may need help. You are unable to pass water while the plug is in place, which means you cannot use it for long, although it is very effective for preventing leakage. It is only used in strenuous activity such as aerobics or running.

Pads and pants

The occlusion devices are only used by a minority of those with bladder problems, younger and more active than most of us. The mainstays of incontinence devices are pads and pants.

Pads

Pads come in all sizes, shapes and styles. Most of them have an absorbent side next to the skin and a waterproof backing. Often there is a strip of adhesive tape on the backing that anchors the pad to your underwear. The pads are either rectangular or shaped like an hourglass, so that they fit comfortably between the legs. This makes a large pad feel less awkward and bulky. Large pads can be difficult to manage and dispose of, so it is better to use smaller ones and change them more often except at night.

Pads are not just stuffing. Most of them contain a highly absorbent powder which is transformed into a gel when it comes in contact with water.

Pads with pouched pants
Pads to wear with pouched pants, so-called marsupial pants, have a waterproof backing in the vulnerable area and a pocket in which to put a pad. A one-way cover to the pocket is intended to keep the skin dry, but it is only effective with light to moderate leakage.

All-in-one pads and pants
This system comes in two types, disposable and non-disposable.

Disposable combined pads and pants are like huge nappies. They are suitable for wearing overnight or with very severe daytime incontinence, for instance from a fistula or false passage. They are also useful when there is leakage from the back passage or double incontinence. They have the maximum absorbency. The snag is their unwieldy size makes them bulky to wear and to carry around and dispose of if you are away from home. They are also expensive but may be supplied free through the NHS.

Non-disposable pants are made of an absorbent material with a built-in pad. They look like ordinary pants at first sight and are washable but the gusset has a waterproof backing. They are only suitable for girls and women who seldom leak much but who want protection 'just in case'. The pad and pants are capable of holding a small teacupful of urine. This means in practice they can only keep the wearer dry with half that amount or less.

Plastic pants

Plastic pants are waterproof and practically airproof. They are definitely not recommended by urologists, gynaecologists, geriatricians and GPs. They are scratchy and uncomfortable and cause sweating and soreness of the skin. They also make an embarrassing crackling noise as you move. The only advantages are that they are cheap, washable and quite effective with wadding inside.

Your skin takes the brunt of frequently being in contact with urine and it is particularly sensitive if you are very senior or bedridden, even temporarily. It adds to the harm if you use talcum powder which is so fine that it can penetrate the skin. Perfumed lotions can cause irritation but a barrier cream such as zinc and castor oil helps to protect the skin in the vital area, as it does for babies.

Clothing

Struggling with pants, tights, jeans and trousers when you are dying to get to the loo can be a lot easier with elasticated waists and Velcro fastenings. The wide legs of French knickers are as accommodating for toileting as an open crotch. Cotton is the least irritating material to have next to the skin. Synthetics dry quicker after washing, but can feel uncomfortable.

Beds and chairs

One nightmare, if you suffer from incontinence, is unknowingly wetting your bed while you are innocently sleeping. You might ruin the mattress and make it smell of urine. The same danger on a smaller scale applies to chairs and cushions. A waterproof mattress cover and breathable materials for protecting pillows, cushions and duvets give you some peace of mind, but mattress covers in particular can make you hot and sweaty. Washable, absorbent bed pads and sheets are convenient. You can lie directly on the bed pad or separated by a one-way absorbent sheet.

This arrangement may be a cause of trouble if you share a double bed. Nightwear can act like a wick if you are using a bed pad. The moisture seeps up your back and chest and makes you cold and clammy, and spreads to anyone near you. The answer is to go to bed starkers or in just a top.

Bed alarm

This is a bed pad that beeps or sounds a buzzer when it comes into contact with water or urine, on exactly the same principle as those used to train small children who don't wake up in response to a full bladder. In either case the object is for the sleepy one to develop an automatic habit of waking just before the leak occurs.

Bedpans, urinals and commodes

Bedpans and urinals

Ordinary bedpans are only needed when you are in hospital or a care home, but small, portable urinals for relieving your bladder anywhere are handy if you are travelling or have difficulty in getting to the toilet quickly when you wake in the morning, or in the night. Urgency is no respecter of convenience.

The usual type is the bottle. For women the neck requires a fit-on extension or the whole bottle may be designed for them. This is the Swan type. There is also a recently introduced urinal that consists of a ring of plastic shaped to fit against a woman's body, and with a handle at the front. A plastic bag with an elasticated opening is slipped over the ring and the urine is passed into this. The bag is removed and sealed until it is convenient to empty it. It may then be thrown away or washed and reused. The big advantage is that it is so small that it can be slipped into a handbag.

Small and larger urinals come in a variety of designs, making travelling and visiting friends well within your compass.

COPING – AIDS AND APPLIANCES

Commodes

These Victorian-sounding pieces of furniture are a godsend to those who cannot easily get to the loo at home, especially at night or when they are alone in the house in the day. Nearly all of them nowadays are made to look like ordinary chairs – square and wooden or Lloyd Loom basket weave. The cheapest is about £40 (in 2003) but these are not always a good buy. There is a wide variation in quality and it is essential, before you buy one, to check that it is right for you. Your feet should both be flat on the floor when you are sitting on it, and it must be designed in a shape that fits you so that none of the urine runs over the brim or splashes.

They are by no means all the same, but most of them, doubling as chairs, have arms and a backrest, and they need a wide base for stability. Some are made to fit over an ordinary toilet – they have wheels and an appropriate top. A wheeled commode is useful to move from one room to another, perhaps for daytime and night.

It is sometimes necessary to use a commode and/or a portable loo temporarily, for instance after a hip operation. The Red Cross Society runs a loan service that lends commodes and other aids to patients who need them. There are around 70 Red Cross outlets scattered over the country that supply health equipment free. Age Concern, the District Continence Advisory Service and branches of the Citizens' Advice Bureau will all help you get what you need. The people who work in them are, almost without exception, caring and glad to help, so there is no need to hesitate about asking for their advice.

12
Coping – medicines

A magic pill to cure incontinence is a pipe dream, but the pharmaceutical industry confidently expects to develop increasingly effective urological drugs over the next ten years. Meanwhile there are medicines already in use that help in controlling the frequency, urgency and urge incontinence caused by detrusor instability. That is when the bladder muscle contracts too often, too forcibly and unpredictably.

Apart from an overactive bladder, there is another situation in which it empties itself at inconvenient times. A *neuropathic bladder* is one in which the nervous controls are no longer working, as a result of damage in childbirth, pelvic surgery, or from a nervous disease affecting the spinal cord or brain, for instance a stroke. Diabetes can have a similar effect.

Reflex incontinence occurs when an overactive detrusor muscle contracts and empties the bladder as soon as it fills, without waiting until it gets the go-ahead from you.

Anticholinergics

Anticholinergic drugs are useful in all these conditions. They act by blocking messages carried by the automatic nerves telling the detrusor muscle to contract and empty the bladder. When the muscle relaxes, the pressure inside the bladder goes down and there is an increase in its capacity.

Oxybutynin (Cystrin, Ditropan), a well-established anticholinergic and the most frequently used, is the standard treatment. It comes in two strengths, 2.5–3 mg and 5 mg. The maximum dose is four tablets a day, using the lower strength if you are elderly. Unfortunately as well as the beneficial effects of reducing frequency and urgency, there are unwanted side-effects on other organs:

- blurred vision
- constipation
- dry mouth
- sore dry eyes

- heartburn
- stomach upset
- palpitations
- nervousness
- fatigue and drowsiness

Occasionally there is an overkill effect from an anticholinergic – it can be too effective. If the detrusor muscle was overstretched in childbirth or is constitutionally weak, the additional effect of the medication in damping down the force of its contractions may tip the balance towards difficulty in passing water. This can lead to retention.

It is risky to take these drugs if you have glaucoma, heart disease or high blood pressure since, if you don't pass as much urine as usual, you retain more fluid in your body, increasing the pressure. This throws an extra strain on the circulation. Ill effects are also likely if you are a man with an enlarged prostate, or are currently taking an antidepressant of the tricyclic group. They have similar properties to the anticholinergics, so you are taking virtually double the dose.

All this sounds off-putting, but, in fact, you are not likely to have more than a couple of the possible side-effects, and they are often slight. Fortunately two new drugs have recently been introduced that are just as effective but have fewer side-effects. Examples include tolteridone (Detrusitol) and propiverine (Detronorm). Sometimes the antidepressant amitriptyline is used instead of a standard anticholinergic because it has milder side-effects, but it is less efficacious.

As well as their use in urgency and frequency in adults, these medicines, both anticholinergics and tricyclic antidepressants, are given to sufferers from bed-wetting, at any age over 12 years. They are also useful to adults who are continent but wake up to urinate too often – nocturia.

Antispasmodics and synthetic hormones

Two other kinds of medication, flavoxate and desmopressin, an antispasmodic and a hormone analogue respectively, modify the symptoms of an unstable bladder.

Flavoxate (Urispas) is the antispasmodic. The dose is a 200 mg tablet three times a day. It is not suitable for children but it is particularly effective in settling the bladder after the slight trauma of catheterization or when there is pain on passing water for any reason. It is useful in situations where anticholinergics are effective and has some of the same side-effects, dry mouth and blurred vision. It can also cause headaches, nausea or diarrhoea and should not be taken in pregnancy. Flavoxate was popular a few years ago but some doubt has since been cast on its efficacy.

Desmopressin (DDAVP, Desmotabs, Desmospray) is a synthetic hormone that supplements the natural hormone, *vasopressin*. It signals to the kidneys to slow down the output of urine, so that the bladder takes longer to fill. Taken at bedtime this can enable you to sleep through the night without having to get up to empty your bladder. It is given to bed-wetters and nocturics. Because fluid is retained in the body, you should not take desmopressin if you have high blood pressure or a weak heart. In this respect it is no better than the anticholinergics.

Desmopressin comes in tablet form or as a measured nasal spray, Desmospray. The possible side-effects are headache, stomach ache and convulsions, and the drug clashes with some antidepressants, tranquillizers and the anti-epileptic, carbamazepine. You cannot take desmopressin continuously because you will have frequency in the day if you take it late in the evening to quieten your bladder for the night. You pass the same volume of water over the 24 hours, whether you take desmopressin or not.

Patricia
Patricia was 50 when her incontinence began interfering with her life. Before that it was only occasional, when she was tired or stressed. Her doctor decided on balance that she had both stress and urge incontinence. He prescribed oxybutynin, and after a few weeks Patricia was delighted to find her symptoms improving. Some months later she began to notice that she was passing water more often, but only in tiny amounts – 25–50 ml. She could not pass more when she tried.

The doctor then diagnosed *retention with overflow* and began treatment by emptying her bladder by catheter. He stopped the oxybutynin which was making matters worse and booked her in for a course of bladder exercises. These continue and she has high hopes of getting control of her water without drugs.

Bethanechol and phenylpropanolamine, used in cold cures, are sometimes thought to help in stress incontinence by increasing the tone or tension in the muscles in the neck of the bladder, which are characteristically weak in this kind of incontinence.

Oestrogen (Premarin, Progynova), the most important female hormone, often plays a secondary role in the treatment of stress incontinence. Unlike urge incontinence, this type seldom responds to medication. Oestrogen can be useful, however, in supporting other treatments, such as drugs, lifestyle or exercises, when there is a shortage of oestrogen because of the menopausal hormonal close-down. Oestrogen enhances the strength and robustness of the sexual organs and others, for instance the skin.

Premarin tablets come in two strengths, 0.625 mg and 1.25 mg. Progynova TS is given in the form of medicated patches applied to an area of skin without hair and below the waist. If you have had a hysterectomy, you can safely take the oestrogen alone, but if you have an intact uterus you have to take a progestogen as well. Hormone replacement therapy (HRT) of the usual combined kind contains oestrogen and a progestogen. Popular examples are Prem-Pak C, Tridestra and Kliofem, all in tablets. Progynova TS comes as a patch and the hormone is absorbed through the skin.

Oestrogen cream (Dienoestral cream) and oestrogen pessaries are both used in vaginitis. They are very effective and do not require progestogen cover.

Diuretics

'Water tablets', or diuretics, stimulate the kidneys to rev up their urine production. They cut down the reabsorption of water.

They are used to reduce the amount of fluid in the body, for instance in high blood pressure, heart and kidney failure, or when there is oedema, a swelling due to excess liquid, seen commonly in swollen ankles.

Osmotic diuretics

Examples are urea and sucrose (sugar), which are not easily reabsorbed. In diabetes there is too much sugar in the blood, and this causes a rapid loss of fluid with an increased output of urine, a characteristic symptom. Diabetes is Greek for prolific flow.

'Loop' diuretics

'Loop' diuretics are the most powerful. They block almost completely the reabsorption of water from the collecting system. Examples are:

- frusemide (Lasix)
- bumetamide (Burinex)

Thiazide diuretics

Thiazide diuretics cause a moderate diuresis (flow of urine), and sometimes a loss of potassium. Examples are:

- cyclopenthiazide (Navidrex)
- bendrofluazide (Aprinox)

'Potassium-sparing' diuretics

'Potassium-sparing' diuretics have a milder effect but are often given in combination with these. Examples are:

- triamterene (Diazide)
- amiloride (Moduretic)

Non-medical diuretics

Non-medical diuretics are the caffeine-containing drinks – tea, coffee, cola, and also alcohol. They are an inadvertent cause of incontinence. Cold weather and a large intake of water or other drinks have a similar effect.

Antibiotics

Any infection of the urinary system, commonly cystitis or urethritis, is liable to cause frequency and sometimes incontinence and when the germ responsible is identified the appropriate antibiotic will usually clear the trouble within 4–5 days. The 'trial and error' method of selecting the antibiotic seems simple, but checking the results of a urine culture is wiser and probably as quick in the end. There is a big choice of medicines, including antibacterials nitrofurantoin (Furadantin) and quinolone (Negram, Ciproxin), the wide-spectrum, all-purpose penicillin, amoxycillin (Amoxil), and an antifungal, nystatin (Nystan).

Trimethoprim is the most popular of the antibiotics for cystitis. It has the great advantage that bacteria do not develop resistance to it and it works well against organisms that are sensitive to it.

Estelle

Estelle disapproved of modern medicine, drug companies and their products. When she developed a sharp attack of cystitis, she refused antibiotics and went to an alternative therapist. In the course of a long, leisurely consultation she was told that the cause of the illness was probably a chill compounded by her liking for curries, strong coffee and bubble baths. Treatment included bed rest, an abundance of herbal infusions, fomentations to the lower abdomen and aromatherapy. The diet focused on vegetable broth, slippery elm gruel, watermelon, carrots, parsnips and garlic. Estelle recovered in ten days, twice as long as it would have taken with an antibiotic, but she had found the experience fulfilling.

Sleeping tablets and anxiolytics

Flurazepam (Dalmane) is a long-acting sleeper and temazepam is short-acting, and those for anxiety such as clorazepate (Tranxene) and diazepam (Valium) all have the effect of damping down signals about how full the bladder is. This can lead to incontinence, especially at night.

Herbal medicine

Herbal medicine is not just a list of herbal remedies, but a complete system of medicine. It was the only system until the nineteenth century, when scientific medicine began to dominate the scene, but in the last ten years it has become increasingly popular, with other forms of alternative therapy.

The triggers to incontinence recognized by herbal practitioners include nervous or emotional strain, coughing and sneezing, or lifting heavy weights. They consider that a 'psychogenic' bladder, that is one sensitive to changes of mood, is an underlying cause of incontinence, but that physical conditions, such as pressure on the bladder, may have an effect.

Other causes put forward by the herbalists are acute stress of any kind, injury or degenerative disease of the spinal cord and some gynaecological disorders, for instance fibroids, ovarian cysts and pelvic inflammatory disease.

Herbal treatments

Urinary astringents are recommended to tighten up the urethral sphincter. These include:

- *teas* – bearberry, American cranesbill, horsetail
- *formula* – for powders, capsules and liquid extracts – cranesbill, horsetail and liquorice; also tinctures in water or honey, for instance a mixture of ehedra, cramp bark and passion flower
- *alternative tinctures* – mixture of ephedra, cramp bark and passion flowers

Other advice

Smoking

Avoid or give up smoking. Researchers in Virginia, USA, report a case control study of 600 women in their forties. It showed that 29 per cent of incontinence was attributable to cigarette smoking.

Sitz baths

Sitz baths are aimed at improving the circulation and nerves of the pelvis, and especially toning up the involuntary muscles of the pelvic floor. Alternate three minutes in a hot bath with one minute in a cold one, repeating the exercise three times, ending with a cold bath. Add 2 pints of infusion of rosemary or camomile to the hot bath – 1 oz (30 g) of fresh or dried flowers and leaves per quart of boiling water.

For pelvic disorders in particular, including incontinence, simmer 1 oz of buchu or bearberry for 20 minutes, strain and dilute with warm water, topping up as necessary. Sit in the bath up to your navel but with your chest, knees and lower legs out of the water. It is easier to achieve this if you sit across the bath, unless you have an antique hipbath. Some health farms have special sitz baths.

A weak bladder in older men can be treated with tincture of thuja – five drops in water three times a day.

Cystitis

Herbalists consider that causes of cystitis include spicy foods, pickles, vinegar and condiments, and also coffee, tea, cola drinks and other stimulants. Alcohol is even worse and meat is regarded as liable to concentrate the urine so that it irritates the lining of the bladder. A chill is thought often to trigger an attack of cystitis.

Herbalists, like traditional doctors, recognize E. coli bacteria migrating from the rectum as a cause of cystitis, but they also blame bath salts and cubes, biological detergents for washing underwear, 'feminine' deodorants and freshener tissues, spermicidal creams, tampons and the contraceptive pill.

Recommendations

Cut out caffeine drinks and alcohol and substitute generous quantities of herbal teas, cranberry juice and barley water to dilute the irritating effect of the uric acid in the urine.

Herbal teas
Herbal teas include:

- cornsilk, marshmallow and elder flowers (marshmallow and cornsilk are both recommended for burning pain on urinating)
- bearberry, couchgrass and buchu (buchu has a reputation as a urinary antiseptic that is particularly effective against E. coli germs, and it is also a stimulant diuretic causing a flow of urine)
- alfalfa
- Maria Treben's tea – a mix of horsetail, lady's mantle, shepherd's purse and yarrow

Aromatherapy
Five drops each of cajeput and juniper in the bath water. Cajeput, from the swamp tea tree, is an antiseptic and an antispasmodic. It is mainly used externally as a liniment for painful joints and toothache.

COPING – MEDICINES

General advice
Bed rest, fluids and warmth.

Fomentations
These require two towels, one wrung out in hot water, the other in cold. The hot one is placed on the middle of the lower abdomen and the genital area for five minutes, alternating with the cold towel for one minute. Continue for half an hour and repeat daily.

Bathing
Hot, soaking baths with juniper and cajeput in the water.

Diet
This is based on plant foods – slippery elm food gruel at most meals, vegetable protein from soya, peas and beans, nuts, and meat substitutes made from processed fungi; polyunsaturated oils, for instance sunflower seed; plenty of raw vegetables and fruit, whole grains. Carrots, garlic and yoghurt are particularly favoured, and vitamins A, B, C and E and zinc as supplements.

Diuretics

Over 300 herbal diuretics are listed, including agrimony, bilberry leaves, bogbean, bugleweed, celery seed, chivers, dandelion, devil's claw, heather flowers, kava kava, lignum vitae, lily of the valley, mullein, vervain, wild carrot and garden nasturtium.

Anti-diuretic

Liquorice root is an anti-diuretic, sometimes prepared as a sweet, for instance Pontefract cakes. Eating too much liquorice can lead to dangerously low levels of potassium in the blood.

13
Coping – surgical operations

Coping with incontinence need not mean pads, plastic pants and near impossible exercises. It is quite different with the help of a surgeon. Her or his approach will be fast, decisive and active – with a high percentage of successes.

Laparoscopic or *keyhole surgery* is revolutionizing surgery and soon nearly all operations, for instance on the bladder, will be done this way. The incisions are tiny and heal quickly and the surgeon sees the view through the laparoscope, a kind of telescope, on a television screen.

Operations for stress incontinence

Colposuspension

Colposuspension, the standard treatment, is a method for supporting the neck of the bladder and urethral sphincter. The operation takes about an hour under a general anaesthetic. Often erstwhile sufferers feel so fit and optimistic afterwards that they tend to overdo it, but it is vital not to put any strain – as from lifting – on the tissues for three months.

Complications

Between 80 and 90 per cent of those who have had a colposuspension are cured. They no longer have 'accidents' and are consequently emotionally and socially much improved. The only major complication is prolapse; and there may, of course, be the kind of complications that can arise with any operation – chest infection, haemorrhage, haematoma (a local collection of blood), wound infection, urinary tract infection, or the accidental injury of adjacent organs, for instance the bladder.

Vaginal sling

This is a simple concept – a support or sling made of a synthetic like Teflon or an autograft of your own connective tissue is slipped under the neck of the bladder and the urethra and attached to the muscle of the abdominal wall. The sling holds the bladder neck in the best position for achieving continence. As with colposuspension, the bladder may be irritable after a sling operation causing frequency and sometimes urgency for days, weeks or even months. It subsides eventually.

Tension-free vaginal tape (TVT)

This recently devised operation is beginning to supersede the ordinary vaginal sling. Its advantage is a shorter recovery period. Two tiny incisions are made just above the pubic bone, about 5 cm from the midline, causing little trauma and rapid healing. Usually a light general anaesthetic is given. It takes about 40 minutes to free the tissues and fit the polypropylene tape under the neck of the bladder.

In 2002 a research study compared colposuspension and TVT, involving 344 women. TVT was as effective as colposuspension in curing incontinence but there were slightly more complications during the operation. Post-operative complications were commoner after colposuspension, and the recovery time was longer.

Needle suspension

Two small incisions are made in the abdomen and a stitch put in each side of the bladder neck to pull it up. It sounds simple, but it takes an hour to perform and requires a general or epidural anaesthetic.

Periurethral injection

This procedure is usually carried out as a day case, but a general anaesthetic is needed. A fine needle is passed up next to the urethra or through it and a bulking agent is injected in the vicinity to cushion the urethra, making it more easily closed. The choice of materials includes redundant fat (your own), animal collagen or synthetics.

The injections are safer but not as effective as the bigger operations. They can be repeated if the effects are too slight or are wearing off.

Artificial urinary sphincter

Since a weak sphincter is a major cause of stress incontinence, the ultimate treatment is to provide a new one, using silicone. It consists of three interlinked parts:

- a cuff fitting round the outlet of the bladder
- a reservoir of urine for controlling the pressure in the cuff
- a pump control

Only a handful of urologists are experienced in this complex surgery.

Operations for urge incontinence

Augmentation cystoplasty
This is also called the clam operation because the bladder is split into two halves like a clam shell. A strip of tissue from the small intestine is sewn in between them, like letting out a garment. It makes the bladder roomier and the pressure inside it lower so that tension and urgency are relieved.

Detrusor myectomy
Part of the muscular coat of the bladder, the detrusor, is removed. This also reduces the pressure inside the bladder.

Bladder reconstruction
A 'new' bladder is fashioned from a length of small intestine, which is 20-odd feet long so can easily be spared. This complicated operation is a treatment of last resort, reserved for young women with aggressive cancer.

Neuromodulation
This is still at an experimental stage. An electrical nerve stimulator, like a heart pacemaker, is implanted near the nerves supplying the bladder. It has proved helpful for those who have become incontinent through a spinal injury paralysing the bladder.

Permanent catheterization
Not a cure but a method for coping, long term, with a *neuropathic* bladder in which the nerve control no longer functions. The catheter may be inserted through the urethra, or by a permanent hole in the abdominal wall above the pubic bones. The latter route is preferable because it is less liable to infection. The urine drains into a bag

strapped to the leg. An option is a catheter with a valve at the end that can be opened periodically, like going to the loo to pass water at intervals. You can learn to change your own catheter if total independence is important to you.

Options in anaesthetics for surgery

1 *General* – you are unconscious and feel nothing. They are usually given as a gas, but may start with a quick-acting injection. You come round gradually and feel sleepy for an hour or two.
2 *Epidural* and *spinal anaesthetics* are given by an injection in the back and prevent your feeling anything below the waist for 3–5 hours. They do not put you to sleep but you are often given a sedative or a light general anaesthetic with the injection.
3 *Local anaesthetics* numb a limited area near the site of the injection. The effect wears off gradually.

14
Training your bladder – exercises

All the continence advisers, nurses and urological consultants swear by the special exercises as the best treatment for incontinence – if only the sufferers would grit their teeth and persist with them. What is even better than improving the dispiriting symptoms of stress and urge incontinence is to avoid them altogether. This, too, is possible if you learn a few important exercises and practise them regularly before you have had any leaks to speak of. For most of us, however, we take the complex action of passing water for granted until we are shocked into paying attention by an 'accident'.

Suddenly we desperately want to be able to keep control.

Basic bladder drill

This is a simple but effective method of building a good toileting routine and checking at an early stage any tendency to leakage. It makes good sense to fill in a three- or five-day *volume and frequency chart*, as a base-line before you begin. You record for each day the number of times you pass water, any episodes of leakage and the total volume passed in the 24 hours. You also need to record the amount you drank. If you drink twice as much you will have to go to the toilet twice as often. Most of us drink about 1.5 litres a day, although some experts recommend 2 litres, and on average we go to the loo 4–8 times in the 24 hours, including once in the night. The volume of urine passed each time is 250–400 ml. There is an early warning when the bladder is getting full, at 200–250 ml, but it can hold 400–600 ml. This is up to age 45, but it becomes less with age. This means the older person has to 'go' more often, since they drink just as much as younger people.

After these preliminaries the drill itself can begin. The aim is to get into the way of passing water at approximately three-hourly intervals without strain or difficulty. You work up to this. Start by emptying your bladder. Then note the time. You must not pass water for the next hour, however strong the urge, but when the hour is up you must do it, whether or not you need to. Repeat this timed urination for a day or two, then increase the interval by five minutes for another few days. It is essential to continue with each interval until you are perfectly comfortable with it. It is better to wet yourself, and then go back to an interval you can manage, than to succumb too easily to the desire to pass water ahead of the appointed time.

This is an example of behaviour therapy – you learn by doing what is wanted and repeating it as often as necessary. There is no limit on how long you may take to achieve your goal. The difficult part is suppressing the desire to urinate as it gets near the end of the self-imposed period. It can be helpful to have something dull and mechanical to do while you are holding your water – cleaning silver or calculating your Income Tax.

Hearing a tap run, or still worse, seeing it, even looking at a picture of Niagara, can intensify the desire to pass water. This is a reminder of how closely your emotions are bound up with your waterworks and a test of how well you are learning to override the impulse to urinate. It is especially relevant if you have the symptoms of frequency and urgency, which can lead on to urge incontinence.

Dorothy Mandelstam of the Disabled Living Foundation, in her comforting, practical book, *Incontinence*, recommends, as part of the bladder drill, stopping the flow in midstream, holding it briefly and then continuing. The object is to practise controlling your bladder. Recently, this ploy has been frowned on by many workers in the field. They say that interrupting the normal flow can disrupt important reflexes. However, it may be done as a one-off to demonstrate what it feels like when the pelvic floor muscles contract. This can be useful to the 30 per cent of women who have only a vague idea about where their pelvic floor is or how to tense its muscles.

Mini bladder drill

You can start this at any time. When you have just passed water, simply note how long it is before you want to do it again, then add five minutes before you do so. Next time add another five minutes, so the interval is ten minutes longer. Go on increasing it until you are unable to last out. Then go back to an interval you can manage until you are confident at that level before going on with the progressive increases.

Double voiding

It is important to empty your bladder completely, especially after intercourse. Stagnant urine in the bladder breeds infection. Emptying it twice running – double voiding – helps to avoid this. After passing water in the usual way, wait a full two minutes, then try again. You usually find a little more urine to pass. Double voiding may help if you are experiencing a temporary difficulty or hesitation in passing water, as may happen after giving birth or an epidural anaesthetic.

Timed voiding

This involves setting an alarm clock and passing water every time it goes off. Choose a comfortable pattern of timing, perhaps every two hours, or before each mealtime. This is particularly helpful in the case of a spinal cord injury when the person cannot feel the appropriate sensations as the bladder fills. It may also help those with other physical or mental disabilities.

Prompted voiding

The prompting is a personal reminder to empty the bladder for someone with Alzheimer's disease or another dementia. Praise for doing what was wanted, in this case passing water, is part of the exercise – performed by the carer.

Posture

It is worth acquiring the habit of sitting on the toilet the way that suits your bladder best. A low toilet is ideal, or else a stool to raise your feet a few inches. Bend forward slightly and place your legs a little apart – having knees and toes neatly together was strictly for the Victorians. Squatting is also good, or standing up and leaning forwards which brings in the gentle force of gravity. These three postures help to keep the neck of the bladder at the right angle.

TRAINING YOUR BLADDER – EXERCISES
Pelvic floor exercises

The important pelvic floor exercises are difficult at first. To start with, unlike the biceps or the calf muscles, you cannot see these muscles in action. They are part of the *perineum*, the area between the inner sides of the tops of the thighs. The pelvic floor is the part that contains muscle and supports the neck of the bladder and the urethra and holds them in position. This is vital for continence. The pelvic floor also supports the rest of the bladder and the vagina.

Before you can exercise them you must locate the pelvic floor muscles in your own body. You start by tensing them, which requires concentration, then you must learn how to use them to squeeze, raise, hold and relax. Try to pull the floor upwards and backwards, then the other way, from the back to the front, but still upwards. A common mistake is to bear down instead – just what you do not want. Postnatal classes in health clubs are excellent for general and tummy exercises but are not often geared to pelvic floor drill.

The best and most convincing way of getting to know your pelvic floor is the vagina test. Place two fingers in your vagina and squeeze them, using the surrounding muscle. You can feel the contraction gently gripping your fingers and the muscle becoming tense. This exercise, applied to your partner's penis, is a very intimate kind of hug, greatly enhancing the pleasure of intercourse.

Contracting your pelvic floor muscles correctly is as delicate and subtle as playing the violin and, equally, calls for a qualified teacher. Five or six 'lessons' are the norm. As with the bladder exercises, pelvic floor exercises require motivation, persistence and patience. The principles are repetition and endurance – doing the exercises over and over – and keeping up the tension for longer and longer. Start by holding each contraction for a count of two and work up.

Exercising your pelvic floor muscles regularly, say five times a day, makes them develop in size as well as strength like the muscles you can see, for instance the pects on a weight-lifter's chest. The extra bulk is especially beneficial in the case of the pelvic floor as it packs in the neck of the bladder, strengthening the closure mechanism by packing it in snugly with muscle. Because these muscles are not on view, you can practise your pelvic floor routine discreetly any time – standing at a bus stop, sitting in a train, lying in the sun or a bath or in bed. For them to have an impact you need to do them five times, five days a week, without fail.

Don't let yourself get disheartened early on. These exercises are truly difficult to master. Mentally they take serious concentration and these unpractised muscles soon tire. Start gently and build them up gradually.

Specific exercises

Exercise 1
Sit on a hard wooden chair with your knees a little apart, leaning forwards with your elbows on your knees. Imagine that you are trying to control imminent diarrhoea on some prestigious occasion. Pull up the pelvic floor generally, using only the pelvic floor muscles themselves. Pull tighter then hold for a count of ten or as long as you can, then slowly relax. Repeat until it comes easily.

Exercise 2
The quick squeeze saves you from leaking when you cough or sneeze. Do a rapid pull-up and quickly let go. This calls into play a different set of muscle fibres from those used for the long, strong effort of Exercise 1. The contraction is immensely powerful but cannot be sustained, like a firework in contrast to a gas burner. Repeat this exercise also, but take a ten-second recovery time between each contraction.

Help in getting the hang of pelvic floor exercises

There is no doubt that it is difficult to control your pelvic floor muscles and to feel them in action, so some methods of making it easier have been worked out.

Perineal stimulation
This involves the use of a *perineometer*, an electrical gadget that is slipped into the vagina. It measures the pressure when you exert the vaginal squeeze on it and reveals any weakness of the pelvic floor muscles, such as commonly underlies stress incontinence. The perineometer can also be used to stimulate these muscles, making

them contract in a passive form of exercise. It is then called a *perineal stimulator*. It causes no pain or side-effects apart from a mild tickling sensation in the vagina when it is in use, but it must not be used if you might be pregnant or have a pacemaker.

The beneficial effects of perineal stimulation in the improvement of stress incontinence are noticeable after a few weeks. A popular method is to insert the stimulator into the vagina for a 10–20-minute spell while relaxing on a bed or sofa in the late evening. Although you may feel practically cured after a month, it is essential to continue with the treatment for a minimum of 3–4 months.

Up to 70 per cent of women who use this method find their incontinence vastly improved after 12 weeks. The muscles are stronger, they can hold each contraction for longer, and do not tire so quickly. However, only 25 per cent of women achieve complete control.

Biofeedback

This method, using a sensor, informs you about the strength of your vaginal squeeze so that you know when you are tensing your pelvic floor muscles effectively, and whether they are getting stronger.

This way you can learn to control them.

Electrical stimulation

This is available in two slightly different types – maximal electrical stimulation (MES) and faradism. It is one of the tools the physiotherapist uses to increase your awareness of your pelvic floor muscles and increase their tone. The apparatus can be used at home once you have learned the way.

Vaginal cones

These are the most popular aid towards training and strengthening the pelvic floor muscles. They are cone-shaped weights that you put into your vagina and hold there. They come in sets of identical size but different weights. Beginners start with a light cone which they can hold with very little effort, and after doing this for two periods of 15 minutes separated by a brief pause, they move on to a heavier cone and so on progressively.

You can buy the cones at most big pharmacies, but it is better to get them through your physiotherapist or continence adviser to be

3× DAY

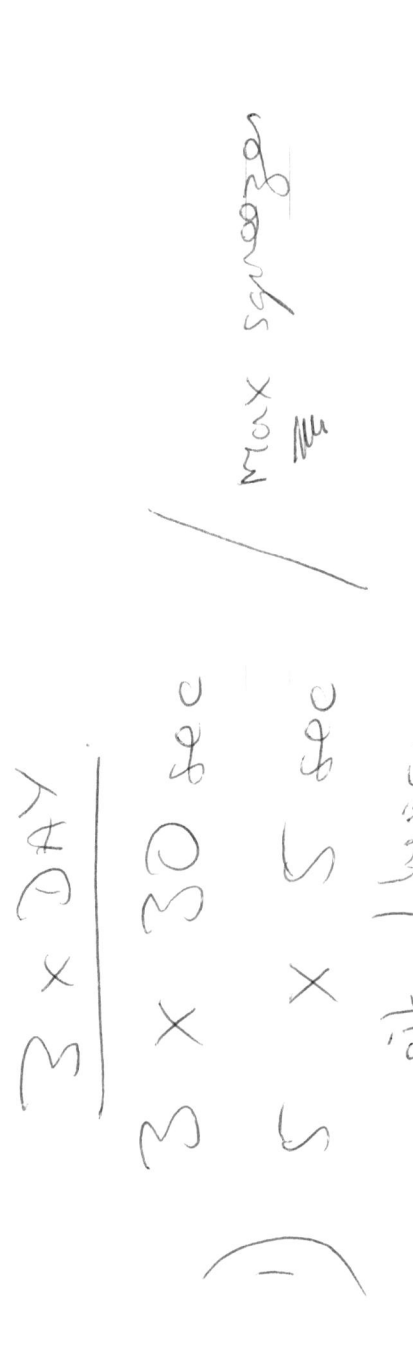

1) 3 × 30 sec
   5 × 5 sec
   1's / by 5's   / Max squeeze

2) Practice 30 sec ↓ stand.

3) Use 30 sec ↑ of doggy #'s / legs

4) Stop test 1× week

TRAINING YOUR BLADDER – EXERCISES

sure of having the right size and weight for you, and of using them correctly. It is important to be scrupulous about washing the cones in soapy water each time you use them, because it is easy to introduce thrush or some other ubiquitous infection into your vagina. This method of exercising your pelvic floor muscles is practical and understandable, but does not suit every case.

15
Faecal incontinence

When someone mentions incontinence we assume they mean the common urinary kind, involuntary leakage of urine, the waste products of metabolism in liquid form. It affects three million people in Britain. No one boasts about it, but still less does anyone reveal the situation if they have *faecal* or *anal* incontinence. The *faeces* or motions comprise the solid waste matter from the digestive system, hence the term *faecal*. The alternative term *anal* refers to the anus, the exit from the gut.

Double incontinence means lack of control of both liquid and solid waste. Faecal incontinence refers to the involuntary passing of motions. It is less common than urinary incontinence, amounting to 90 sufferers in 10,000 compared with 600. It is far more distressing, not only for the sufferer but also for the family. It is the ultimate turn-off, however blameless the sufferer.

Some old people whose muscles, including those of the urethral and anal sphincters, have become weak and lax from age, can leak a little from the back passage as well as the front, soiling their underwear.

> *Ada*
> Ada, 84, was in this embarrassing situation occasionally, but only when she had taken a laxative and her motions were loose.

Another 'normal' reason for such accidents is an attack of diarrhoea. The anal sphincter is not designed to hold back fluid. Babies, of course, are doubly incontinent, but as their nervous system develops, they gain control. The bowels are mastered first – as early as 15 months for some. It is a matter of maturity and training. At the other end of life, time is not on our side. A tendency to leak from the bowel requires an overhaul of the diet, so that it contains enough fluid and fibre to prevent rock-hard stools, but not so much that they are runny. Large, all-in-one pads and pants, like giant-size nappies, are effective but expensive, unless you get them free through the NHS. They are inconveniently bulky and difficult to dispose of discreetly.

FAECAL INCONTINENCE

Although faecal incontinence is not common, there is a string of possible causes for it and it can affect people of any age and in any mental state.

Joyce
Joyce was 27 when she happily became pregnant. She was small, just under 5 ft, while baby Joe was a big strapping fellow of 8 lb-plus when he was born. In addition he obstinately refused to stay in the normal head-down position in the uterus, preferring to arrive bottom first – a breech birth with forceps. By the time he had made the 4-inch journey into the world both Joe and his mother were exhausted but apparently unharmed. It was only during the recovery period that it emerged that Joyce's pelvic floor had been badly damaged. She had no control over bladder or bowels, a disastrous situation, especially at her age.

A battery of electrophysiological tests showed that fortunately most of the damage involved the pelvic floor muscles rather than the nerves. A series of operations repaired the muscles. This, plus physiotherapy and endless patience, led to a great improvement over the next six months.

Mandy
Mandy was a beautiful baby but she had spina bifida, one of several congenital malformations in the anorectal region that interfere with the nervous control of the bowels. Surgery is the main treatment.

Molly
Molly had neglected her bowels for years, never giving them enough fruit and fibre to get a grip on, but preferring to indulge in her favourite diet of crisps, chocolate and cheese in a bun, washed down with coke. With such an unbalanced diet she was chronically constipated and regularly took a strong chemical purgative. This emptied her bowel but left it unresponsive to the normal stimulus of food for several days. By then she felt she needed the laxative again and a vicious circle arose.

Molly developed *faecal impaction*. A hard motion blocked the colon except for a little liquid faeces that escaped round the sides. Molly's bowel was gently cleared with enemas and from then her diet was revolutionized to include fruit, vegetables, bran and whole grain with plenty of water. Her lifestyle was altered to include a 40-minute walk or an exercise class three times a week. It took four or five months before these changes began to have the desired effect.

Margaret
Margaret had piles (haemorrhoids). They had been brought on by frequent straining and now they were preventing the anal sphincter from working properly by getting in the way. A minor operation disposed of the haemorrhoids, but, like Molly, Margaret required a healthier diet and exercise to tone up her muscles all over.

Prolapse of the rectum

Prolapse of the rectum means that a fold of the lining of the rectum is forced out through the anus during a muscular effort to empty the bowel. It produces similar symptoms to external haemorrhoids, has a similar cause – frequent straining to pass a motion. It also requires simple surgery and a more bowel-friendly lifestyle. This involves a dietary review, to include 2 litres of water daily. The waterworks require this to function at their best. The bowels need plenty of fibre in fruit, vegetables, whole grain cereals and bran. The abdominal muscles are toned up by such exercises as bicycling on your back and sit-ups. A regular time-table for meals, exercises and toileting is helpful in developing good habits.

The nerves controlling the bowel, like those running the urinary system, comprise two types, autonomic or involuntary, which work automatically through reflexes, and the voluntary kind that come under the will. They all arise from the lower end of the spinal cord. Damage to the involuntary component causes constipation while damage to the voluntary type causes faecal incontinence. The muscles involved in continence of the motions are the important group in the pelvic floor and the puborectalis, the sling muscle that supports the neck of the bladder among other parts.

FAECAL INCONTINENCE

Kirsty
Kirsty was a near-anorexic. She felt that if her food passed through quickly it would not put any weight on her. That had meant taking increasing doses first of a herbal laxative, but then of a chemical purge – until her colon would not respond any more. Currently she is coping as best she can with enemas three times a week. Hopefully, when her bowel has been rested and she has been given some weeks of healthy living, including a nourishing diet with plenty of carbohydrate as well as protein, she can be rehabilitated into regular bowel habits.

The management of faecal incontinence is difficult, but some medicines can be helpful. Loperamide (Imodium) and diphenoxylate (Lomotil) both act by reducing the bulk of the motions. The main lesson with this type of incontinence, once the initial blockage is cleared, is to avoid overuse of laxatives, especially the chemical stimulants such as sodium picosulphate (Picolax), and to deal with constipation by increasing the amount of fruit, vegetables and bran in the diet, and drinking plenty of water. A good ploy is to have a tumbler of hot water first thing in the morning and ensure a fluid intake of 2 litres daily.

To start with replace any chemical purges with an osmotic type like magnesium sulphate (Citromag), which draws fluid into the bowel, then progress to bulk laxatives such as ispaghula husk (Fybogel) and finally to manage with foods such as figs, prunes and bran. A glycerol suppository provides an occasional rescue package, or a simple enema does no harm.

16
Thoughts and feelings – the psychological aspect

Incontinence isn't painful or disfiguring, but it accounts for more misery and humiliation than any other common disorder. It causes emotional suffering and damage to the quality of life. The feelings that flood the sufferer's mind are shame, guilt and an ever-present fear of public disgrace. This is the stuff of nightmare – a nightmare that can become real at any time.

Last Sunday I went to church to sing carols with the children and I could not help noticing that three chairs in the back row each had a circular patch of discolouration in the middle of the seat. I felt a stab of sympathy for the three ladies from the rest home who always sat there. Their bladders had let them down and, sadly, no one had told them that there were ways of escaping the constant risk of such tell-tale evidence. It is estimated that 48 per cent of incontinence sufferers get no help because they hide the problem.

Proper management guarantees improvement, if not outright cure, but at best this takes weeks, maybe months, after you have screwed up your courage to ask for help. Meanwhile there are desperately unhappy feelings to contend with – anxiety, guilt and clinical depression.

Anxiety

Anxiety is natural in the circumstances. If you were driving your car and found that you could no longer control its speed or direction, it would be surprising if you were not afraid. That is how it is when you lose control of your water. Your mind is in turmoil and your heart rate quickens when you think of what might happen and where – for instance when you are shopping in the high street. Your muscles get tense and trembly so that you can hardly walk. Anxiety itself stimulates the bladder and you have an acute desire to pass water, even if you visited the loo five minutes ago.

Non-stop worry about your bladder leaves you exhausted but you

THOUGHTS AND FEELINGS – THE PSYCHOLOGICAL ASPECT

look perfectly well so no one guesses what torments you are suffering – will you be able to sit through the concert without disrupting a whole row of the audience by going to the toilet in the middle of the performance, or worse still, not getting there. Chronic anxiety can be assuaged by two means. First by talking, explaining your fears to someone sympathetic. This blunts the edge of it. Then you are ready for the cognitive approach.

This means a therapist guiding what you say so that you find that you are arguing yourself out of the frightening feeling that disaster is waiting round the next corner. Replace it with positive thoughts such as the determination to learn and then conscientiously practise the bladder control exercises. Their effectiveness has been proven, given time. Simultaneously, take up a new interest to give your mind some distraction – studying art history, playing the guitar, crocheting a beret, joining a choir, etc.

You may not have the patience for the slow-but-sure approach unless you see some results. You need an instant boost, but do not abandon the talk-and-practise method. It is worth latching on to anything you have already gained from it, but invest also in the immediate calming effect of a small dose of an anxiolytic (*anx* means anxiety, *lytic* breaking down). The best known is diazepam (Valium), but others are alprazolam (Xanax) or buspirone (Buspar), which belongs to a different drug family. As well as softening the edge of anxiety, an anxiolytic will help you sleep.

Insomnia

Insomnia is a distressing symptom of anxiety. Just when you think you have dealt with all the problems of the day and you are tired to the bone, your mind and your body refuse to relax. The medication blurs your anxious thinking and helps you to drift away into slumber, but it loses its effect if you take it for more than a week or two. Stop the tablets as soon as you are sleeping reasonably well and use bodily exercise for mental and physical relaxation, leaving your concentration unimpaired.

THOUGHTS AND FEELINGS – THE PSYCHOLOGICAL ASPECT
Guilt

Guilt comes next in frequency to anxiety. Of course this is not reasonable. You know that you are not incontinent on purpose but you cannot help feeling ashamed, as though you were. Guilt is cousin to depression and dates back to your early childhood, when the blackest days were those when you had been naughty, in your parents' eyes. You felt a total outcast because you were bad; the sun did not shine for you. Before you were two years old you had learned that 'clean and dry' equates with 'good' and that your urine and motions are 'dirty' except when they are in a potty, when they are suddenly, miraculously good.

You can try arguing against your feeling of guilt, but instead of its subsiding you may slide into a clinical depressive illness. This presents with a feeling of hopelessness and a draining away of vitality. You sleep but you wake unrefreshed, and much too early. Incontinence can be a symptom, a kind of weeping.

While clinical depression may respond to cognitive psychotherapy, there is often a chemical component to the illness, when it is better treated with antidepressants. The most popular of these is fluoxetine (Prozac), one of a group called SSRIs – selective serotonin reuptake inhibitors. These increase the availability of serotonin, a chemical messenger that lifts mood.

For lesser degrees of depression a down-to-earth way of dealing with low spirits brought on by incontinence is to join a support group. A problem shared is a problem halved, or at least put into perspective. It is reassuring to discover that other people have the same difficulties as you. A sharing of horror stories brings out the funny side, and an exchange of tips on how to cope. Awkward situations include staying at a friend's house, going for a long hike with a group, sitting through an opera with an enthusiast, or attending a funeral in a bladder-chilling east wind.

The pundits insist that you should not pass water when your bladder is only half full, 'to be on the safe side'. But as a matter of practicality, if you have to be on view for 2–3 hours because of some important social occasion, it is wise to start off with an empty bladder, and to avoid having a bloodstream full of caffeine-laden fluids like coffee. If you use pads it makes sense to wear one of generous size, and to take two spares with you. You are less likely to leak if you are 100 per cent prepared.

When you have got through the major event, revert to the training programme of holding your water for a definite period and gradually edging it up to the limit. An incontinence problem makes every sortie away from home into a project. Pessimists or the prudent prepare for eventualities by finding out in advance about toilet facilities, and if necessary pack a bottle-type loo in your hand luggage.

Quality of life

There is no doubt that incontinence impairs your quality of life, if you let it. For a start you have to cut down on such shareable minor pleasures as coffee, tea, fizzy drinks, alcohol and cigarettes – they all stimulate the bladder. However, most of the restrictions depend on the psychological reaction to incontinence. A sad case, quoted by Jane Smith in the excellent book, *Keeping Control*, describes a woman who did not go out for nine years for fear of wetting the car seat.

Travel is one of the main casualties, from a shopping trip into town or a safari across Africa. It means having to find out about, and plan ahead round, the availability of toilet facilities. You do not want to be caught short at the supermarket checkout, or waiting for your flight to be called at the airport. Abroad you may have language difficulties and pray for a pictorial clue to indicate a loo. Fortunately these are becoming more prevalent.

Mainline stations present a series of obstacles. Finding the toilets is the first, then struggling up and down stairs with luggage is added before reaching them. Women with toddlers can have particular difficulties. The cubicles are not big enough for mother, child and buggy. The essential is to allow twice as long as you had expected.

Treats and celebrations you would once have enjoyed can turn out to be ordeals.

Restaurant and other meals out are a common, harmless treat unless something 'goes down the wrong way' and you have a fit of coughing and choking. This is a severe test of the strength of the quick-acting muscles of the urethral sphincter.

Entertainment in the shape of theatres, concerts, cinema or opera pose problems if the performance lasts longer than the time-span

THOUGHTS AND FEELINGS – THE PSYCHOLOGICAL ASPECT

your bladder will tolerate. If you are always ducking out when friends invite you to join them, they will stop asking you. To keep your relationships in good repair it is essential to say 'Yes' to most invitations and work out how afterwards.

Relationships with family, friends and lovers are the golden thread that enhances your quality of life.

Sex and romance are arguably man's and woman's top experience, but incontinence means, at a practical level, that intimacy can be a dodgy situation. Intercourse incontinence, affecting younger lovers, is embarrassing – be sure to start with an empty bladder (see p. 37). There may be a physical barrier to intercourse if you are using a vaginal pessary for a prolapsed uterus; the situation is compounded by the age-related shortening of the vagina. It is a matter of remembering to take the pessary out in advance. Or intercourse may be agony if you have the vaginitis that results from a menopausal lack of oestrogen. This can easily be treated by an oestrogen cream, but that involves preparing at least a week ahead, or use lashings of KY jelly in emergency.

It may be difficult to feel romantic when your plumbing system is liable to leaks, but it is worth making an effort. Sex is a physical and a psychological tonic, good for warding off the effects of stress or feeling old. Go for it.

17
Cystitis

Cystitis, like all the other 'itises', is an inflammation, in this case of the bladder. It may also include *urethritis*, inflammation of the urethra.

If you are a woman you stand a high chance of having at least one attack of cystitis in your lifetime. We are much more susceptible to this bothersome disorder than men. This is largely because the female urethra, linking the bladder to the outside world, is less than a quarter the length of that in men. Germs from the back passage, which may cause infection in the bladder, do not have so far to travel.

With so much suffering in silence about problems below the waist it is difficult to assess the true figures for the prevalence of cystitis. Some authorities estimate that one in five women will suffer from it at some time, while others put it at one in three or, vaguely, as 'most' women. It can occur at any age but there are two peak age spans, 30–40 and 55–65. While, over the last few years, the numbers have been falling slightly for the older group, among younger women cystitis has been escalating recently, in line with sexually transmitted diseases. One reason is that intercourse starts at an earlier age and is more frequent than it was five years ago, increasing the risk of infection or irritation.

Lynda
Lynda began having attacks of cystitis when she was 24, shortly after Jeff had moved in. It started off, the first time, with a tummy-ache low down which she thought was a period pain, and then she noticed that she was having to go to the toilet much more often than usual. It did not sting at first but it felt uncomfortable, but she did not think it worth going to the doctor about. It was then that she had an accident to her left hand and the wound became infected.

The doctor prescribed a five-day course of the antibiotic amoxycillin, and while her hand healed her abdominal ache and her frequency subsided too. It had not occurred to Lynda that these symptoms were also due to an infection – bacterial cystitis.

CYSTITIS

Symptoms

While an attack of cystitis usually lasts less than a week, it is painful and unpleasant, and, most importantly, it introduces the blight of incontinence to sufferers, often for the first time. Leakage is likely to be of the urge variety and it may continue long after the cystitis is better. Urge incontinence involves an overwhelming impulse to pass water. When the delicate membrane lining the bladder is red, swollen and inflamed, it is irritated by the urine and tries to get rid of it by passing it every few minutes. It stings or burns each time although there may only be a few drops each time. This is called *dysuria* and it is a characteristic symptom of cystitis.

Another symptom is a dull, continuous pain low in the abdomen, just above the pubic bones at the front – *suprapubic* pain. The sore, inflamed bladder lining often bleeds, colouring the urine pink and sometimes producing clots. There is often a high temperature, the heat of battle, as the body's defences fight off invading bacteria, and elderly people in particular, when they are feverish, may become temporarily confused.

Causes of cystitis

- Infection by bacteria, most often *Escherichia coli* (*E. coli*), which have migrated from the colon via the back passage. Several activities increase the risk, for instance sexual intercourse, horse riding or cycling. Irritation in the area can also be caused by tight jeans, ill-fitting underwear and thongs, which have recently become popular. Bubble baths, perfumed soap and body lotions, bath cubes, deodorants and after-bath splashes all contribute. Talcum powder, although soothing on dry areas, is so fine that it works its way into moist skin and is the worst of all. Creams and ointments, including some advertised as especially intended for 'feminine hygiene', can also irritate this sensitive area, especially during a period.
- Vaginitis, causing irritation and soreness with thinning of the tissues, affects those past the menopause who are feeling the effect of a reduced supply of oestrogen.
- A stone in the bladder, catheterization for any reason, or even an ill-fitting tampon can cause irritation, as can certain methods of

contraception, for instance the diaphragm, or a spermicidal cream. Some of these may also cause difficulty in emptying the bladder.
- Cigarettes.
- Incomplete emptying of the bladder leading to stagnation.
- Finally, in the early months of pregnancy pressure from the uterus crowding the bladder within the pelvis.

The symptoms of bacterial cystitis can all be produced by these diverse causes of irritation. As many as 20–30 per cent of women with these symptoms have no infection at all on investigation.

Recurrent cystitis

Three per cent of women suffering from cystitis will have repeated attacks. Three or more attacks a year qualify as recurrent. These can become a regular feature in a woman's life, and she may get to sense 12 hours in advance when an attack is coming. Any of the risk factors for irritation and cystitis listed above may be responsible for recurrences, but especially incomplete emptying of the bladder. Frequent non-specific triggers are being 'run down', stressed, tired or having a minor illness, like a cold. It is useful to look for links between particular events or situations and an attack.

Ploys to reduce the risk of cystitis

- Try to drink 2 litres of water or water-based drinks every day, omitting the fizzy type, and 1.5 litres is a minimum. This helps by diluting the urine and washing out the bladder and the surrounding area of perineum.
- Drink cranberry juice. The berries contain condensed tannins that prevent E. coli becoming attached to the cells of the urinary system.
- Barley water, sodium bicarbonate or potassium permanganate in water may be used in the absence of cranberry juice. They act by making the urine more alkaline and unattractive to the organisms.
- Empty your bladder completely every time, leaving no stagnant urine.
- Wipe your bottom from front to back after a bowel action or urinating – a bidet is ideal, but lukewarm sponging is sufficient.

- Do not have a really hot bath – it can set off the inflammation.
- If you wear a pad, wash whenever you change it.
- Pass water and wash the area after sex.
- Avoid getting thoroughly chilled, especially your back.

If cystitis only develops after intercourse, it may be prevented by a single dose of an antibiotic, for instance trimethoprim, before or immediately afterwards. Another avoidance tactic is to take one dose of antibiotic daily indefinitely in the hope that this will prevent an infection taking hold.

Interstitial cystitis

This is a non-stop disorder with the key symptoms of frequency, urgency, suprapubic pain, and often incontinence. The frequency may run at once every ten minutes, driving the sufferer to despair. The suprapubic pain, low in the abdomen, is continuous but not sharp. *Haematuria*, blood in the urine, commonly occurs, an alarm signal you must never ignore.

Interstitial cystitis may be preceded by a series of attacks of the ordinary bacterial or irritation-based cystitis and is liable to be misdiagnosed as recurrent cystitis, but it is a different type of illness. The cause is unknown, but it is not bacterial, nor due to the other common causes of cystitis and not associated with sexual activity. Fortunately the condition is quite rare by statistical standards, but it affects around 400,000 people, mainly women, worldwide, 95 per cent of them white. Once established, it continues relentlessly.

One theory is that it is an autoimmune disease, one in which the body's immune system turns on its own cells as though they were enemy aliens. One clue is that there is an unusually large number of *mast* cells in the bladder wall. These enhance the production of histamine, and are associated with the symptoms of inflammation – redness, swelling, pain and stiffness.

A sample of the lining of the bladder in this form of cystitis shows that it is thickened and inflamed with areas of fibrosis or scar tissue. The result is that it is stiff and inflexible and its capacity is reduced. This is an additional reason for the frequency. The lining readily bleeds and is extra sensitive as it is inflamed. It is agonizingly painful to drink cranberry juice, which is good for the other forms of cystitis, but too acid for the supersensitive bladder of interstitial cystitis.

The majority of sufferers are middle-aged but the illness can strike at any age from about 20. In the last few years there has been an increase among the 20–30 year olds in particular. Often it is several years before the correct diagnosis is made. The investigations that clinch the matter are cystoscopy – looking inside the bladder with a cystoscope; and biopsy – examining a sample of the affected tissue under the microscope.

Treatment

Treatment is hampered by our not knowing the cause of the illness, nor even what triggers it. The choice includes:

- long-term antibiotic treatment for three months minimum
- aspirin, paracetamol and other anti-inflammatory drugs
- steroids in severe cases, for instance prednisolone
- bladder antiseptics by mouth, for instance nitrofurantoin (Furadantin)
- antihistamines, such as chlorpheniramine (Piriton)
- antidepressants, for instance imipramine (Tofranil), if for no other reason than that many sufferers are depressed by their symptoms

These drugs are given in the hope but not the certainty that one of them will help. If the situation becomes truly unbearable there is the last ditch treatment of cystectomy, surgical removal of the bladder and the fashioning of a replacement from a redundant piece from the small intestine. Only a handful of surgeons have the skill to carry out this operation.

Children

A urinary infection affects only 1 per cent of boys under 11, but three times as many girls. Most are affected in the first 12 months. Up to half of them have a *vesico-ureteric reflux* – flowing backwards of the urine from the bladder up the ureter towards the kidney. This carries the risk of pyelonephritis, kidney infection. Because of the danger of permanent damage to the kidneys, all children with a urinary infection are thoroughly investigated. Ultrasound is used in babies plus a kidney-ureter-bladder X-ray later.

Surgical treatment may be required if there are repeated infections or reflux persists. Parents need to ensure that the child does not become constipated and has plenty of water to drink. A small, regular dose of an antibiotic may break the cycle of recovery and re-infection. The possibility of sexual abuse must be borne in mind as a possible cause of recurrent infection.

Pyelonephritis

This is the most important complication of cystitis, carrying the risk of permanent scarring of the kidney and leading to kidney failure. It can develop from cystitis by the backward spread, up the ureter, of the bacteria in the urine. The characteristic symptoms are malaise – feeling really ill – a high temperature, and pain in the loin, the part of the back lying over the kidney, usually on one side more than the other.

The diagnosis is made by dipstick urinalysis. A spatula coated with chemicals is dipped into a specimen of urine. It allows for two tests – the leucocyte esterase test which detects pus cells in the urine, and the nitrite test which indicates the presence of bacteria. They change nitrates into nitrites.

In serious illness a sample of urine, midstream to avoid contamination, is examined under the microscope. Pus cells and bacteria can be identified, confirming the dipstick test. Tests are carried out at the same time to find out to which antibiotics the bacteria are sensitive. X-ray of the urinary system, kidneys, bladder and ureters, and an ultrasound examination, show up stones and other abnormalities in the upper part of the urinary tract. These include strictures of the urethra, narrow places resulting from previous infection with scarring, and in men, pressure from an enlarged prostate gland.

Bacteria attach themselves to the lining of the system to do their damage and one of the beneficial effects of cranberry juice is to prevent this. Urinary infection is a particular risk in pregnancy, and pyelonephritis is a serious complication. Before the advent of antibiotics it was responsible for a number of maternal deaths. It is important to diagnose and treat the illness promptly.

There is another rare, but dangerous, illness which is more of a risk for those who suffer from chronic cystitis.

Bladder cancer

Bladder cancer, unusually for urinary problems, is mainly a man's disease, often because of the work they do. In fact it is the fourth commonest cancer in men, after prostate, lung and colon cancers. The chemicals that can lead to bladder cancer include the aniline dyes and benzidine, and occupations that can be risky are dry cleaning, painting and decorating, and car mechanics. Cigarette smoking increases the risk tenfold, or the presence of a stone. Both of these irritate the lining of the bladder.

The first symptom of the illness is usually haematuria, blood in the water without pain, unlike the haematuria that may occur in cystitis. The symptoms may begin with frequency, urgency and dysuria, pain on passing water, as with simple cystitis. Pain in the loin is the give-away, but often develops later when one of the ureters has been blocked by the tumour. Treatment is surgical. Fortunately the benign forms of bladder problems are many times more likely, especially for women.

Elizabeth

Elizabeth's was a typical bladder disorder. She was a widow of 60. She had 'always' had what she called a weak bladder. She suffered from bouts of cystitis 4–5 times a year, when she was afraid that she would not get to the loo in time, although usually she managed it. It seemed that no sooner had she recovered from one attack of cystitis than she was starting the next. There was hardly any time when she was not afraid of wetting herself, and her life was spoilt. Although antibiotics helped they only cleared the problem up temporarily.

Her doctor put her through a series of investigations including an ultrasound examination of her bladder. The reason for Elizabeth's repeated infections was a stone in her bladder. That in turn was partly due to the incomplete emptying of her bladder, so

CYSTITIS

that there was always some residual urine in it. For the stone itself Elizabeth went to a centre in a nearby hospital where they had all the facilities for dealing with stones. For self-help she increased the amount of water she drank and did some exercises to tone up the muscles in her urinary system.

18
Problems with passing water

If incontinence is your bugbear you might think difficulty in urinating would be welcome; but it involves a load of problems and a particular type of incontinence – overflow.

Acute retention of urine

There is a complete, usually abrupt, loss of the ability to pass water, accompanied by severe discomfort to agonizing pain. Sometimes there have been warning symptoms beforehand, for example transient stoppages or a weakening of the stream of urine so that it degenerates into a slow dribble. In other cases it happens out of the blue. It affects men more often than women since the commonest cause is pressure on the urethra by the prostate. This gland hugs the outlet at the base of the bladder and has a natural propensity to enlarge from middle age onwards. By the age of 80 most men are suffering from symptoms connected with their prostate.

Although women seldom suffer from acute retention, they are not immune. Blockage can be caused by pressure from a fibroid, a non-malignant tumour of the uterus. The immediate treatment is the same in either sex – draining off the trapped urine through a catheter. Usually it is passed into the bladder via the urethra, but if this has caused problems in the past the catheter is inserted through an incision in the abdomen, just above the pubic bone – *suprapubic* catheterization. After the acute situation has been relieved the underlying cause is sought and the treatment chosen accordingly.

Chronic retention of urine

Again men predominate among the sufferers, but not so markedly as in acute retention. The chronic condition creeps up insidiously. It may first show itself with *nocturnal enuresis*, wetting the bed at night. The bladder is not emptied completely, leaving a reduced capacity. This can fill up quickly and overflow during sleep – the same result but with a different cause from childhood enuresis, which is due to immaturity.

After catheterization there is often a spontaneous impulse to pass water by the normal route. This is called *post-obstruction diuresis.*

Symptoms

The symptoms of chronic retention include:

- Hesitancy – you feel you need to pass water but when you get to the toilet there is a delay of several moments before the flow begins. When it does, the stream is weak and comes in fits and starts, finally petering out in a dribble. When it finally comes to a halt you are conscious that you have not emptied your bladder completely. Sometimes only about 25 ml is voided. The amount left in the bladder is the *residual urine*. It may be as much as 200–300 ml, enough to fill a large mug. This stagnant pool is a breeding place for infection and facilitates the formation of stones.
- Stretching of the bladder with excess urine means that it rises above the edge of the pubic bone at the lower border of the abdomen, and may be felt through the abdominal wall.
- Burning pain on passing water, *dysuria*, is mainly due to infection.
- *Strangury*, acute pain with retention, which is almost exclusively a male problem.
- Haematuria, blood in the urine.
- Frequency because of the reduced capacity of the bladder.
- Straining to pass water because of irregular, inefficient contractions of the detrusor muscle, due to having been overstretched.
- Urgency, sometimes urge incontinence, also due to unstable detrusor activity.

Causes of retention

- *Benign hyperplasia of the prostate.* Like a fibroid in a woman, this tumour is harmless in itself but may cause problems by pressure on the surrounding tissues, in this case the outflow from the bladder.
- *Prostatic cancer* causes similar obstruction, but is less common – the symptom to alert you to this possibility is blood in the urine.

PROBLEMS WITH PASSING WATER

- *Constipation* with rock-hard waste matter is a simple cause of obstruction.
- *Stricture of the urethra* is a narrowing of the canal due to previous infection and scarring.
- *Cystitis* and *urethritis*.
- A *fibroid* or occasionally an *ovarian cyst* may press on the bladder neck.
- *Stone disease* is often associated with residual urine and infection. At 3 per cent it is much less common in the UK than in other developed and developing countries. Treatment is essential because, apart from obstruction, it makes the sufferer extra vulnerable to infection and haematuria and even to bladder cancer. It requires expensive high-tech equipment that is only available in a few dedicated centres.
- *Bladder neck dyssynergia* is a form of malfunction in which the relaxation of the urethral sphincter does not synchronize with the contractions of the detrusor muscle of the bladder. An X-ray that outlines the urinary system with a contrast medium in the urine will show if, instead of being released, some urine is trapped in the bladder by this mistiming.
- *Pain on passing water* can also lead to retention. If you understandably avoid the act for too long, your mind cuts it out of your repertoire and you have to spend time relearning it. Post-operative pain, especially after surgery for incontinence, is notorious for causing retention, similar to childbirth and also usually temporary.
- *Childbirth*. Difficulty in passing water often follows having a baby, especially with an epidural anaesthetic which knocks out the nerve supply to the bladder temporarily. After an epidural, a catheter is left in place for 12 hours or until normal sensation returns. A long or complicated labour or the use of forceps increases the risk of damage to nerves and muscles.

Avril

Avril was having her first baby at 21. She was generally fit but had a *scoliosis*, a sideways curve in her spine. This made it awkward to give her an epidural injection, so she settled for old-fashioned gas and air with the birth. Drowsiness came and went, depending on how much nitrous oxide she inhaled, but the pain was controlled. She was congratulating herself on having sailed through the whole affair smoothly and produced a beautiful baby boy (nearly 7 lb) until she found she could not pass water.

She tried harder, and panicked when nothing happened. The sister talked her out of her anxiety, gave her a big mug of tea, naturally laced with the diuretic, caffeine (a bladder stimulant), and turned both wash-basin taps full on. Suddenly the sphincter relaxed and the difficulty was over. Sometimes a warm bath soothes and relaxes the bladder, or an electric pad warming the abdomen and back.

Incomplete emptying, detrusor malfunctioning, retention and overflow incontinence can all be caused by loss of control due to neurological disease or injury to the nervous system:

- cerebrovascular disease, that is furring up, or bleeding due to high blood pressure, of the arteries to the brain, sometimes causing a stroke (*cerebrovascular accident or CVA*)
- Alzheimer's disease
- Parkinson's disease
- multiple sclerosis
- damage to the frontal lobe of the brain
- tumour or injury to the spinal cord
- spina bifida
- slipped disc with a trapped nerve

Treatment

Transurethral prostatectomy
Transurethral prostatectomy, the surgical removal of the prostate through the urethra, is the standard treatment for difficulty in urinating due to the most frequent cause – benign hyperplasia of the prostate. This operation usually works well but fairly common complications are loss of libido, faulty ejaculation and impotence. There may be detrusor instability and incontinence. These effects are fewer with a suprapubic prostatectomy, that is via an incision in the abdomen, but it is a bigger operation. Other types of difficulty with urinating require different management.

Treatment is essential in cases of stone, detrusor overactivity or back pressure on the kidneys from the bladder. It is also needed for infection, haematuria, copious residual urine, or unmanageable incontinence.

In other situations there is a range of possible ploys:

- watchful waiting or 'wait-and-see'
- surgery
- indoramin (Doralese), an alpha-blocking drug
- microwave or laser ablation of the prostate

Claire

Claire's problem was William. He was ten years older than she was, and at 60 was having occasional, but increasing trouble with unexpected episodes of urgent incontinence. It seemed that they occurred most frequently on special social occasions – dinners, receptions and the like. William was always taken by surprise but Claire was the one most acutely embarrassed. In the end she persuaded him to ask for advice, and the doctor examined him carefully, including, to William's disgust, a rectal examination or PR (per rectum). The doctor was able to feel a smooth, painless, slightly enlarged prostate gland.

The suggestion of surgery horrified William. He had heard that a prostatectomy would mean the end of his sex life, something he could not contemplate. However, he did agree to take the tablets, and listened glumly to the doctor's advice to cut down drastically his social drinking of alcohol, and the five cups of strong tea he had at breakfast. When he drank less at night he was not as thirsty in the morning.

William was not cured but when he kept to the regimen his propensity for leakage became manageable.

19
Lifestyle

Since, if you are a sufferer, incontinence impinges on every aspect of your life, it makes good sense to organize your lifestyle accordingly. Step 1 is to take stock.

Questionnaire

Start with a score of 100 and take off 10 for every 'No', leaving you with a percentage score of how healthy you are.

1. Are you generally satisfied with your energy level?
2. Can you hold a conversation while you are walking up a hill?
3. Is your weight within 8 lb (4 kg) either way of your ideal weight? (See Table 1.)
4. Do you cope without any regular medication, including laxatives or mild pain-killers?
5. Have you stopped smoking, if you ever did, more than five years ago?
6. Do you limit yourself to two alcoholic drinks a day? A drink is a single measure of whisky or gin, a small sherry, a small glass of wine or half a pint of lager, beer or cider.
7. Do you limit your intake of chips, chocolate, fries, dips and spreads to very occasionally, and avoid pies, pastries, cakes and chocolate?
8. Do you go for greens, salads and fruit at 2–3 meals a day?
9. Can you enjoy what you consider a really good meal?
10. Do you sleep well without having to get up more than once in the night?

If your score is less than 50 per cent take action now.

If you are aged 50-plus it is high time to take incontinence precautions or treatment.

If you are under 80, you are at a good age for achieving results. The exercises become harder and slower if you do not start them until after the big eight-0 although they are still worth doing.

LIFESTYLE

Symptoms of incontinence anxiety that impinge on your lifestyle

- Cutting down on fluids – concentrated urine irritates the bladder and makes it vulnerable to cystitis – and incontinence.
- 'Loo-hopping' – taking every opportunity of visiting the toilet whenever you go out, even just shopping, visiting a friend, or having a meal, and of course, the moment you get home, whether you need to or not, or the last time was less than half-an-hour ago. Some people visiting for example an exhibition, a theatre, a petrol station or a sports centre make checking the loos their first priority. Others have mental if not paper maps of the whereabouts of all the toilets in town. Supermarkets in general are disappointing since many have no facilities. Loo-hopping increases your anxiety and trains your bladder the wrong way – never allowing you to forget your bladder.
- The 'in case' syndrome – always going to the toilet before going out, before and after a meal or chancing to pass a loo sign. Mothers often urge their children to go to the cloakroom, not at the signal from their bladder but because it is a convenient moment. This disrupts normal communication between bladder and brain.
- Straining to pass the last drop of urine. You get to feel your bladder should be emptied even when it is less than half full.
- Allowing constipation to develop so that you have to strain to pass a motion, damaging the vital pelvic floor muscles. Constipation is mainly a matter of diet and exercise, which you can adjust yourself.
- Giving up activities you enjoy for fear of needing the toilet at an inconvenient time, for instance a fun outing by coach or in a friend's car.
- Playing nine holes of golf instead of 18 because you are afraid of going too far from the clubhouse.
- Missing out on active sports such as squash, tennis, football (for either sex) or athletics. Wearing a pad for the game, with a spare in the locker room, is usually all you need if the leaking is confined to vigorous activity.

LIFESTYLE

Acceptable weights for women

Height		Weight (average)	
metres	*inches*	*kilograms*	*pounds*
1.45	57 (4'9")	46	102 (7 st 4 lb)
1.48	58 (4'10")	46.5	103 (7 st 5 lb)
1.50	59 (4'11")	47	104 (7 st 6 lb)
1.52	60 (5')	48.5	107 (7 st 9 lb)
1.54	60½ (5'½")	49.5	110 (7 st 12 lb)
1.56	61 (5'1")	50.4	112 (8 st)
1.58	62 (5'2")	51.3	114 (8 st 2 lb)
1.60	63 (5'3")	52.6	117 (8 st 5 lb)
1.62	63½ (5'3½")	54	120 (8 st 8 lb)
1.64	64½ (5'4½")	55.4	123 (8 st 11 lb)
1.66	65 (5'5")	56.8	126 (9 st)
1.68	66 (5'6")	58.1	129 (9 st 3 lb)
1.70	67 (5'7")	60	133 (9 st 7 lb)
1.72	67½ (5'7½")	61.3	136 (9 st 10 lb)
1.74	68½ (5'8½")	62.6	139 (9 st 13 lb)
1.76	69 (5'9")	64	142 (10 st 2 lb)
1.78	70 (5'10")	65.3	145 (10 st 5 lb)

Acceptable range: from 4 kg (8½ lb) below average to 7 kg (15 lb) above average.

Table 1: Acceptable weights for women and men. Figures based on British and American standards.

- Avoiding social occasions such as weddings, parties and funerals.
- Wearing skirts for speedy access, when you would prefer jeans.
- Drenching yourself in perfume in case you smell of urine although normal hygiene with a daily bath abolishes the possibility. Fresh urine does not smell unless there is an infection present.

LIFESTYLE

Acceptable weights for men

Height		Weight (average)	
metres	*inches*	*kilograms*	*pounds*
1.58	62 (5'2")	55.8	124 (8 st 12 lb)
1.60	63 (5'3")	57.6	128 (9 st 2 lb)
1.62	63½ (5'3½")	58.6	130 (9 st 4 lb)
1.64	64½ (5'4½")	59.6	132 (9 st 6 lb)
1.66	65 (5'5")	60.6	135 (9 st 9 lb)
1.68	66 (5'6")	61.7	137 (9 st 11 lb)
1.70	67 (5'7")	63.5	141 (10 st 1 lb)
1.72	67½ (5'7½")	65	144 (10 st 4 lb)
1.74	68½ (5'8½")	66.5	148 (10 st 8 lb)
1.76	69 (5'9")	68	151 (10 st 11 lb)
1.78	70 (5'10")	69.4	154 (11 st)
1.80	71 (5'11")	71	158 (11 st 4 lb)
1.82	71½ (5'11½")	72.6	161 (11 st 7 lb)
1.84	72 (6')	74.2	165 (11 st 11 lb)
1.86	73 (6'1")	75.8	168 (12 st)
1.88	74 (6'2")	77.6	172 (12 st 4 lb)
1.90	75 (6'3")	79.3	176 (12 st 8 lb)
1.92	75½ (6'4½")	81	180 (12st 12 lb)

Acceptable range: from 5 kg (11 lb) below average to 8 kg (17 lb) above average.

The danger of ducking out of doing things with other people is that in the end they don't invite you. Overhaul your lifestyle before you turn into a recluse.

General health

The most feared illnesses – cancer, heart disease and stroke – can all be avoided to some degree by healthy living.

Risk factors for the big three which are under your control include:

LIFESTYLE

- too much fatty food
- alcoholic binges
- smoking
- lack of exercise – you are only 2 per cent brain, 98 per cent muscle and bone
- too few fruit and vegetables
- overweight, especially the 'apple' shape in which the waist is bigger than the hips. In the safer, more feminine 'pear' shape fat is concentrated below the navel and on the thighs and bottom.

The good news is that the number of strokes is down by a quarter in the West, and the risk of cancer reduced by a third if you follow a healthy diet. You are more likely to find the most troublesome problems are not life-threatening, for example period pains, arthritis, migraine, or – of course – incontinence.

Tired all the time (TATT)

Do you get six hours' sleep? Sleepers and tranquillizers may help you sleep, but at the cost of low energy in the day, and in some people enuresis in the night. Fresh air and exercise and a later bedtime are the safest ploys. Other health problems – chest or heart – may drain your energy, or could you be anaemic? It can creep up silently, for instance from blood loss due to heavy periods round the menopause, piles, the medicines for arthritis, or a poor diet. Anaemia is likely to be the iron-deficiency type, and six weeks on iron tablets will set you up. Anxiety and depression can also make you feel tired 'when I've done nothing'. Overweight is naturally tiring – it is like carrying two suitcases round all day (see pp. 116, 132).

Skin problems

The area most affected by incontinence is the perineum, the part between your legs where the urethra, vagina and anus open. Redness is a warning about a pad rubbing or sensitivity to a detergent used for laundry, bath salts, perfumed soap or talcum powder. The best preventive of sore skin is washing or bathing in lukewarm water morning and evening and, when you change a pad, rinsing well if you use a little mild soap. Baby lotion can be massaged in gently but adult creams and lotions are best avoided. The exception is a barrier cream if it is difficult to keep the skin dry.

Any broken skin needs keeping clean, and protection from pressure or rubbing. If you are over 60 you may have the dry soreness of vaginitis, due to lack of oestrogen. This calls for oestrogen by mouth, for instance Premarin, or a vaginal cream, Dienoestrol. The cream has the advantage that you do not need to take a progestogen with it.

Chronic cough

Smokers, asthma sufferers and those with chronic bronchitis put a sudden, sharp pressure on the pelvic floor muscles many times a day and sometimes at night. The rise in pressure from each cough is transmitted from the abdomen to the bladder and the urethra, but if the pelvic floor muscles are weak, for instance due to childbirth, they may not be able to support the bladder neck, and the mechanism for closing the sphincter may not be strong enough on its own. It is important to try every means to improve the cough from giving up cigarettes, to anti-asthmatics, flu jabs and antibiotics. Cough suppressants, such as pholcodine linctus, are useful to quieten the cough centre but can also suppress messages from the bladder when it needs to urinate.

Pelvic floor exercises, including the Kegel type, are the most important long-term treatment for a chronic cough, and overweight needs correcting.

Edna

Edna was 70 and as sprightly as a teenager. She enjoyed her food but was not overweight. She was never bored but always on the go. Her one weakness was her liking for cigarettes – something non-fattening that did not need cooking which she could offer to her friends. A lot of them did not smoke, but Edna herself only had five a day, after meals and in the evening. Her little dry cough did not trouble her until she got flu.

This was in December. What with Christmas, she felt she was too busy to go to the surgery for a flu injection. That left her breathing system unprotected while it was disabled for 15 minutes five times a day, for each of her smokes. Edna succumbed to the virus during a cold snap and developed influenzal pneumonia. Antibiotics did not help and the bouts of coughing strained her pelvic floor muscles.

It was the beginning of her incontinence. Her chest recovered but the incontinence continued, with leaks when she made the slightest effort. She is now struggling with pelvic floor exercises and has given up cigarettes for good.

Constipation

Constipation is extremely common, particularly with today's easy-to-eat foods, based on processed carbohydrate. Without adequate amounts of fibre there is not enough stimulus to the muscles of the bowel. An adult requires 30 g of fibre daily, the amount in 13 Shredded Wheat biscuits. All-Bran, dried prunes, figs and apricots, the skins of jacket potatoes, bananas and large quantities of green vegetables, plums and citrus fruits are all rich in fibre. Their disadvantage is that they tend to cause bloating (see p. 113).

Overweight

The three top causes of ongoing excessive strain on your pelvic floor muscles are constipation, coughing and overweight, all of them related to your lifestyle. Overweight is the commonest and the dreaded middle-aged spread is often mistakenly regarded as inevitable. It is true that your metabolism gradually slows down with increasing age. Between the ages of 25 and 65 it slows by 5 per cent, even if you are eating the same amount as before and taking just as much exercise. In fact you probably do less physically and eat richer food in the menopausal years.

You already know what you should do – take in fewer calories and spend more of them on regular exercise sessions from swimming to aerobics. Five minutes climbing stairs burns twice as many calories as jogging, while walking instead of riding mounts up to miles each week. Always be the one to fetch something from upstairs or the kitchen and take up badminton, table tennis, orienteering, dancing, bowls – something you have not done before. But don't lift heavy weights, or help to push a car up a hill – your pelvic floor will suffer.

Addiction

Hopefully you are not hooked on cocaine or heroin, but what about coffee, chocolate, alcohol, laxatives, analgesics, cigarettes or just food? It takes four months to douse out a craving so prepare for a

Headaches

Persistent or frequent headaches spoil your quality of life. They come in several flavours – migrainous, tension type or anxiety/depression. They are hardly ever caused by eye problems but are often triggered by your lifestyle. Working in a stuffy, polluted atmosphere on one hand or exposure to an icy east wind on the other can bring on the pain. Irregular meals also put you at risk. Skipping a meal means a dip in your blood sugar and that causes headaches. Women are more sensitive to hypoglycaemia than men (*hypo* means under or less, *glyc* sugar, *aem* blood). Treatment must be prompt but is simple: a Marie biscuit and a handful of raisins. Prevention means spreading small meals out through the day, with no mega gaps.

Sherry, red wine, port and beer all contain *tyrosine*, which makes the arteries in the brain contract and cause migraine in some people. Mature Cheddar or Stilton cheese also contain tyrosine and can have the same effect. You learn from personal experience what to avoid. Dry white wine in moderation is usually safe, but drink plenty of water afterwards. Lack of water-based fluid will, in itself, cause a headache, as in the dehydration of a hangover. Hangovers are bad news on several counts for anyone with a tendency to leakage – alcohol irritates the lining of the bladder locally, and stimulates the kidneys to produce more urine.

Strong filter coffee is another drink that should not figure in your lifestyle. It is a powerful diuretic and, like all stimulants, can also produce a headache or stomach-ache. Go for tea or decaff instead and remember that you need 1.5–2 litres of water every day. A nightmare meal for your waterworks starts with sherry and continues with red meat and red wine. Ripe Stilton follows dessert, together with brandy or port and cigarettes or a cigar. You don't bother to drink any water . . .

The treatment for a headache involves a breath of cool fresh air and such simple analgesics as paracetamol or soluble aspirin. Paracetamol is kinder to your lining, but aspirin is marginally more effective. For definite migraine there is a new group of medicines.

Sumatriptan (Imigran) is the longest established but is not suitable for those under 18 or over 65.

Worrying is a potent cause of tension headache. Try to put your problems to bed before you go.

Insomnia

There is no health risk with insomnia, but the bleak misery of trying to get to sleep when all the rest of humanity is snoring snugly needs circumventing before it develops into a habit. There are more don'ts than do's to break the vicious circle of a bad night then a sleep in the day 'to make up' followed by a repeat performance again and again. Never doze in the day if you aim to sleep at night. Beware especially of the after lunch dip in concentration and the lullaby effect of evening television. Set a cooking alarm to wake yourself up if you tend to drop off by mistake during the evening.

Don't go to bed at nursery hours. Even if you get off to sleep at 9.30 or 10 p.m. you are likely to wake up in the small hours, with no more sleep in you and have to lie there until the world wakes up. Lying in bed and not sleeping does nothing for you. Just as your mind and body learn the wrong sleep/wake rhythm if you go to bed too early, so it is counter-productive to 'lie in' after a poor night's sleep. It is better to get up when you wake up if it is 5 a.m. or later.

Some insomniacs thrive on a small alcoholic nightcap and this is probably better than taking a sleeping tablet. Alcohol is metabolized quite quickly but the tablets do not switch off their action when the clock says that it is getting-up time. The drug is gradually cleared from your bloodstream during the day by the liver cells but it may make you into a zombie during the early part. The other inconvenience is that it may be too effective in the night, so that you are too heavily asleep to respond to the message from your bladder that it is full.

Arthritis

This wear and tear disorder affects everyone sooner or later. By the age of 35, 66 per cent of men and 44 per cent of women show the signs of the condition in an X-ray of the lower back. The disparity is probably because men do more of the heavy work and play more violent sport. You do not see female footballers hurling themselves

LIFESTYLE

to the ground regardless. Why so many of us get joint problems is because of the way we walk, balanced vertically on two limbs, throwing enormous strain on our hips, knees and back. You can feel them complaining the morning after a vigorous work-out, or an afternoon's gardening. They are sure to be stiff and may be painful if they have become inflamed. This condition can be short-lived and acute or become chronic. Injuries and operations affecting the joints, their extra heavy use as in the case of athletes, and the added burden of obesity all increase the chances of chronic osteoarthritis.

This is a common cause of incontinence, especially in the night. Because of stiff, awkward movements, especially when you first get out of bed, you may not get to the loo in time. As you get older there is a shorter time lag between the moment when you realize that you need to empty your bladder and the flow beginning.

Treatment

Treatment usually starts with medication, a non-steroidal anti-inflammatory drug or NSAID. Examples are ibuprofen (Nurofen, Brufen) and the more recent celecoxib (Celebrex). These work well, but joint replacement, especially of a hip or knee, is well-established as the best answer to this painful disability when the medication is no longer effective. Hip replacement is particularly successful, with a minimum of complications.

Back pain is wearying and depressing, as though you were carrying a heavy burden all the time and sometimes it irritates the bladder indirectly.

Prevention
- Do not overwork your joints and muscles.
- Avoid sudden muscular efforts – damaging to the pelvic floor and your lower spine.
- Do gentle stretching exercises only, or yoga, if you have recently put an extra strain on your joints.

Diabetes

This comes in two types, one affecting mainly the under-forties and the other, far commoner and on the increase, sneaking up in middle age. It tends to run in families and affect mainly those with a sweet tooth who have been plump for some years. From 50 onwards, but

LIFESTYLE

especially in the sixties and seventies, the body begins to lose control of its carbohydrate metabolism. It cannot deal with starchy and sugary foods – bread, potatoes and pasta, and all the sweet treats in the form of cakes, buns and pastries. This leads to there being too much sugar in blood, which makes you thirsty, a characteristic of the disorder.

Naturally you drink a lot and that leads to frequency and sometimes incontinence. This may be the first indication of the illness. The complications of diabetes can be serious – high blood pressure, serious eye problems, and skin infections especially affecting the feet. It is essential to have a blood test and if that indicates diabetes, to start treatment without delay.

Psychological suffering

What is so unfair about emotional pain is that there is nothing to show, so you do not get the sympathy and support you deserve. Yet the effects of incontinence are to siphon off your self-confidence and make you feel illogically guilty, and chronically anxious about keeping dry. The symptoms of anxiety can be vaguely physical, including headache, racing heart, loss of appetite, poor sleep and fatigue.

The worst thing to do is use alcohol or a tranquillizer hoping it will make you feel better. Either of these will sap your spirit, but the company of friends and a cup of tea may help.

Relaxation exercise

This can be used when you are stressed, anxious or miserable.

- Flop into a comfortable chair or lie flat on the bed or the floor.
- Take three deep breaths and close your eyes.
- Scrunch up your toes, then relax them slowly.
- Point your toes then use your calf muscles to pull them towards you.
- Hold, then leave go.
- Bend your knees towards your chest, then slowly straighten them.
- Straighten your knees as far as they will go, hold and relax.
- Pull in your tummy, hold the relax.
- Tense then relax your pelvic floor.
- Press your buttocks together for a few seconds.

LIFESTYLE

- Make tight fists of your hands then spread your fingers.
- Tense your arms and shrug your shoulders, then relax.
- Screw up your eyes and think of someone or some place you care about.

Get up and splash your face with cold water – and come alive.

20
Outline of a day

Set your alarm 15 minutes early, to give you a good start to the day.

Programme

1 On waking, while you are still horizontal, do half a dozen pelvic floor pull-ups (see p. pp, 84–5).
2 Then quickly get up. Lingering in bed is counter-productive – any enthusiasm for the new day leaches out.
3 Once you have got up and been to the loo throw on a few clothes.
4 Reward yourself with a hot cup of tea and a Marie or Rich Tea biscuit unless you are on a super-strict slimming jag. Some people prefer plain hot water for their first drink of the day – healthy, but it is an acquired taste.
5 Run through the following mini exercise session.

Limbering

Stretch in all directions – arms, legs and back, for starters.

Do 6–10 each of the following exercises:

- Lift your left knee to a right angle then replace your foot and swing your leg forwards and backwards.
- Repeat with the right knee and leg.
- Swing each leg out to the side, then behind you.
- Touch your toes.
- Lie on your back on the floor or on your bed.
- Pull in your tummy for a count of four or more.
- Bicycle your legs.
- Lift each leg in turn to the vertical.
- Rotate your ankles clockwise and anticlockwise.

OUTLINE OF A DAY

- Sit up then lower yourself gently onto your back, no hands (try to do each exercise ten times).
- Grab your toes, knees straight.
- Stand on tiptoe.
- Hold onto a chair-back and bend your knees until you are in a squatting position. Come up again.
- Sit on a hard wooden chair and pull your left then your right knee up to your chest.
- Replace your legs for the normal sitting position, then stand and sit. Repeat 20 times (this is a very useful exercise, it saves you from an undignified struggle getting out of a soft, low chair).
- Clench your bottom muscles.
- Pelvic floor drill (see p. 84).

---

6 Now you are limbered up feed the cat, dog and birds and prepare breakfast for yourself and any family living at home.
7 Breakfast is the most important meal of the day. Cereals, toast and marmalade provide instant energy, while egg, ham, cheese or sardines give you sustained nourishment. The meal plus the hot drink will set off the gastrocolic reflex at a convenient time to empty your bowels.
8 Pass water and note the present time, and the time for the next voiding. This can be up to three hours later if your bladder is already well trained. Otherwise allow the longest period you think you can manage, hopefully half an hour or upwards. Try not to go to the loo before this. If you easily succeed with this add five minutes to the interval next time (see p. 82).
9 Plan your day round the inescapables – your outside job and/or the tasks you must undertake at home and with the children.
10 Build into this breaks for fresh air and tea, coffee or a herbal beverage, preferably with a companion. Breaks can range from five to 15 minutes and you need one every hour-and-a-half to keep time with your body clock. Meals come at roughly three-hour intervals – block off 30 minutes or an hour for each, to include a stint of exercise.
11 Hour-long exercise sessions, in the gym or the pool or just walking, are essential 2–3 times in the week, but at weekends feel free.

12 Always walk instead of riding in a bus or car whenever you can, and look upon climbing stairs as an opportunity for first-class exercise.

Evenings

The serious part of the day is over. You enter a different phase of living at a less frenetic pace in which friends and family and your own personal interests have top priority. TV, music, books and hobbies come into their own. You may enjoy computer games, surfing the net or following a course of study. Workaholics find something related to their job. Going out in the evenings is a must for the young, but a less frequent pleasure for those with a more settled life. Drinks with friends, either alcohol or coffee, can have an unwelcome effect on your bladder and you may not know where the toilet is.

The evening meal

Unlike breakfast when you are fuelling up for the day ahead with one eye on the clock, the emphasis for the evening meal is on pleasure and relaxation. Other people to share it rate tops, but if you are on your own there is surrogate company and plenty of entertainment on the box or the radio; or you can read your book.

This meal should be leisurely and enjoyable, but not a big one. A full stomach puts pressure on your bladder and it also makes you thirsty. A lot to drink of any kind is unwise at this time. You do not want to be disturbed in an hour or two by the need to get up and empty your bladder. Another disadvantage to a sumptuous supper is that when you are asleep and doing nothing more active than turning over, your digestion can process and absorb every single calorie. This revs up any tendency to put on unwanted weight.

Winding down to bedtime

A regular ritual gets you into the mood for slipping easily into sleep. In summer take an evening walk and in winter do a few free standing exercises to loosen up your muscles. Either way finish by toning up your pelvic floor muscles, their final session for the day. Review your day. Was there a balance between work and play, rest and exercise and social contacts? Did you have healthy meals and the recommended 1.5–2 litres of fluid? And what are your priorities for tomorrow? Your mental computer can be preparing for this overnight.

Bath-time
An evening bath cleanses mind and body from the detritus of the day and is soothing to the spirit. If you are a lark rather than an owl, you will probably prefer a morning tub to wash away sleepiness and leave you sparkling fresh. A shower in the morning is especially enlivening. Hygiene is particularly important to you if you have a waterworks weakness, so don't skimp it – enjoy it.

Nightcap (optional)
A *small* milky drink rounds off the day comfortably for some of us. Horlicks has been shown, in a scientifically conducted trial, to induce longer, deeper, more peaceful sleep. A short alcoholic drink is good for switching off the problems of your waking life, but the effect wears off in two hours and you can wake up fully alert.

Bedtime
The most popular time for hitting the hay or putting your head on the pillow is around 11 p.m., when the best TV shows are over. If you try to go to sleep too early, even if you manage to get off satisfactorily, you are likely to wake up far too soon, fully refreshed, and have tedious hours waiting for everyone else. Going to bed too late can leave you fagged out by noon the next day. The best method is to run your life like a dance – to a rhythm.

> *Peter and Josephine*
> Like Jack Sprat and his wife, Peter and Josephine were incompatible, but not in their taste in food. Instead they had incompatible body clocks. Peter was always early and Josephine always lagging behind, until halfway through the evening when he would be yawning and she was getting into her stride. As in the case of the Sprats they worked out a *modus vivendi*. On working days Peter got up first. He had his shower and made tea, emptied the rubbish, and had breakfast ready by the time Josephine struggled downstairs. In the evening Peter was fagged out and fell into a chair with a drink while Josephine rustled up

the supper. She was also in charge of any entertaining, but Peter did the washing up next morning.

It worked better to go with the natural flow than trying to force uniformity. Both partners appreciated periods of privacy. Josephine liked to do her exercises in the morning and sort out any incontinence problems when she changed her clothes for the evening.

21
Nourishment and repair

We need food not just as fuel but also for mending parts of the body that have been injured or worn. Women are at particular risk, for instance of damage during labour to the pelvic floor and the ligaments that hold the bladder in place. The enormous loss of first-class protein needed to make a baby needs replenishing but many women in their forties and fifties have never fully recovered from pregnancy and child-bearing. Top quality nourishment is also vital for carrying out repairs of the inevitable damage incurred during the months-long strain and stretching of pregnancy and the birth.

This may not be all. Breast-feeding gives the baby a Rolls Royce nutritional start but at the cost of further inroads on the mother's reserves. Added to the depletion following childbirth, there is an ongoing call on her energies from the load of physical work caused by a baby. Women, especially those who have borne children, need an extra good, properly balanced diet. They often miss out.

All new mothers are short of time and deadly tired (though happy), and there is an overwhelming temptation to fill up on snacks instead of having nourishing, but not necessarily fattening, meals. Mothers are likely to skimp meat dishes that need cooking because they are too much effort and take too long. The traditional 'meat and two veg' is an excellent provider of the vital protein and complex carbohydrate (plant) foods needed for building and repair, together with a steady supply of energy. What comes to a busy woman's mind instead is something quick she can eat in her hand, washed down by cups of caffeine-laden coffee or tea.

Cakes, buns, biscuits and chocolate involve no more effort than it takes to peel off the wrapper. Their taste is addictive. The basic ingredients are sugar and fat, the least desirable elements for a healthy diet. No better is the most popular savoury – a packet of crisps, made largely of fat and salt and liable to have a deleterious effect on blood pressure. Mothers are not the only ones to neglect their own nutrition. Quite apart from the long-term effects of having babies, a modern woman's life is complex and demanding. Often she has to pack two careers into the same 24-hour day. One is running a home with its multiple ramifications; the other is keeping her end up in the highly competitive outside world.

Greta
Greta coped with her accustomed efficiency when, added to her stressful job as a Ward Sister at the cottage hospital, she had baby Jeremy to collect from the crèche, plus the shopping, the cleaning and the cooking. She managed to scramble through giving Jeremy his evening feed, his bath and his story-time before Neville came in tired and hungry from a day's work and an hour's commute. By then Greta was 'bone tired', as she put it, and although she usually managed to make a meal for Neville she was too exhausted to do more than pick at her own plate.

It was understandable that her after-baby leakiness should go on and on. She had no time for the two hours feet up in the day, as recommended, and standing up put a continuing pressure on her pelvic floor. The slightest extra pressure on her bladder, even stooping to tie her shoelaces, was too much for the urethral sphincter and pelvic floor muscles, weakened by the recent pregnancy and labour and having had no chance to recover. It was when her GP was on holiday and his place was taken by a woman locum that her life was reorganized. Greta negotiated a transfer to a sitting down job and shared the home chores with Neville who discovered a hidden talent for cooking. The change that made the biggest difference was the exercise plan, with a specialist nurse who helped Greta to learn the knack of exercising her pelvic floor muscles. She could do the drill at odd moments in the day, and found, after 4–5 weeks, that her incontinence was gradually improving.

Women like Greta somehow manage to look after everyone else, but often have many of their own meals standing up in the kitchen. They deserve something better than these snatched, scrappy snacks. They need a good, balanced diet. This is not as simple as it seems since no two experts think exactly alike on what that is.

The food gurus of Britain and the United States, supported by their governments, each provide guidelines for the populace. The Americans are more generous in their recommendations. For instance, their standard for an alcoholic drink is 12 g of alcohol compared with 8 g in Britain, but more is not better when obesity is the foremost nutritional disease in the affluent West.

The British 'healthy diet' guidelines

1 Top comes enjoyment – try different foods, so that you do not miss a treat. Except for special medical reasons, nothing is absolutely barred.
2 Variety is healthy.
3 Be sparing with salt.
4 Eat the right amount to stay at the right weight (see p. 112). Fats and oils give you more than twice as many calories weight for weight as proteins and carbohydrates.
5 Be generous to yourself with starch and fibre – bread, potatoes, rice and cereals, and the pea and bean family.
6 Go for lots of fruit and vegetables. They may have a protective effect against chronic diseases like cancer.
7 Be sparing with fats, especially animal fat, and sugary foods and drinks.
8 Alcohol – no more than 3–4 units a day for men, 2–3 for women.

Dietary 'guidelines for Americans'

1 Total fat – not more than 30 per cent of the daily calorie count:
 – saturated fat – less than 10 per cent of the count
 – eat fish regularly for omega-3 polyunsaturates.
2 30 minutes or more of moderate exercise daily.
3 Balance food versus exercise.
4 Moderation in the intake of sugar, salt and alcohol, and low in fat.
5 One alcoholic drink a day for women and two for men count as moderate.
6 Five-plus helpings of fruit, especially citrus, and vegetables, especially green and yellow, daily.
7 Six or more servings of bread, cereals and legumes daily.

There is not much to choose between these two standard guides.

Suggestions for a general purpose diet

Never miss breakfast – some slimmers cut this meal out but that is counter-productive – it is what you eat in the evening that can lead to weight gain. You have all night to digest it, so not a calorie is lost.

The diet

Early morning tea, coffee or herb tea, and semi-sweet biscuit if desired.

Breakfasts

Ring the changes with one of these:

1 Porridge, semi-skimmed milk and stewed fruit, or an apple or orange.
2 Muesli, semi-skimmed milk, one slice of toast, spread and marmalade, apple.
3 Grilled tomato, mushroom and/or baked beans on toast.
4 Shredded Wheat, All-Bran or Weetabix and a handful of sultanas or prunes, semi-skimmed milk.
5 Three fresh fruits, wholemeal roll and honey.
6 Half a grapefruit, boiled, poached or scrambled egg with toast and spread.
7 Slice of grilled ham or lean bacon with tomato and toast.
8 Yoghurt, fresh fruit, two slices of toast and cheese spread.
9 Sardine on toast, banana.
10 Dried prunes or apricots (cooked) with oat bran porridge or Ready Brek.

Drink tea, coffee or hot chocolate.

Midmorning

Decaffeinated coffee or tea, semi-sweet biscuit if desired or a piece of fruit.

Lunches

1 Jacket potato with cottage cheese, ham, fish or baked beans filling, salad, fruit juice.
2 Vegetable soup, brown roll, cheese, apple.
3 Meat, ham, egg, fish 2–4 oz (30–100 g) with vegetables (green

NOURISHMENT AND REPAIR

and yellow vegetables) and potato, tap or spring water.
4 Wholemeal sandwich with protein filling as in 3, with salad or celery, juice.
5 Chicken or tofu, broccoli and sweetcorn, bread roll, water.

Optional coffee, decaffeinated.

Teatime

Tea, plain scone and spread, or fresh fruit in season.

Suppers or dinners

Starters (optional)
Melon. Crudités. Fruit juice. Avocado. Clear soup.

Main course
1 Stir-fried chicken and mixed vegetables.
2 Curried beef, rice, vegetables.
3 Macaroni cheese, peppers and tomatoes.
4 Grilled fish, peas, potatoes.
5 Baked ham and leeks or broccoli.

Water, tap or mineral, or glass of wine.

Second course
1 Fruit sorbet or fresh fruit.
2 2-inch cube of cheese, water biscuits.
3 Apple pie.
4 Ice-cream.

Coffee – decaffeinated usually.

The total daily calorie count should be 1,900–2,000 kcals for women, 1,800 after age 60, and 500 kcals more for men.

Do not hurry your meals, listen to the radio or read if you are on your own, and do not go over your worries or have a disagreement at mealtimes.

Diets for special circumstances

High fibre diet

To avoid constipation – one of the contributors to incontinence.

1 *On waking*. Two cups of hot tea to wake up the bowel.
2 *Breakfast*. Half a grapefruit, an orange or 4–5 prunes, porridge or

NOURISHMENT AND REPAIR

All-Bran, slice of wholemeal toast with spread and chunky marmalade, coffee or tea, decaffeinated, two cups.
3 *Midmorning.* Piece of fruit, decaffeinated coffee or mineral water.
4 *Lunch.* Vegetable or lentil soup, wholemeal sandwich with ham, egg or cheese, fresh fruit, juice or water, decaffeinated coffee.
5 *Tea.* Tea, coffee or juice, 1–2 oatcakes.
6 *Supper.* Jacket potato including skin with meat, tuna or cheese filling, salad, stewed rhubarb with half a banana sliced up in it or baked apple, mineral water or small glass of wine.
7 *Bedtime.* Digestive biscuit and hot skimmed milk or camomile tea.

For a high fibre diet avoid white bread, pastry, cake, rice and pasta.

Baked beans, lentils, peas and green beans, and natural bran, provide plenty of fibre but may cause bloating. Adjust the amounts accordingly.

Make sure of adequate fluid – 1.5–2 litres (2.5–3.5 pints) daily.

Reducing diet

Extra fat increases the pressure on the bladder, especially when you bend forwards, and is a major contributor to stress incontinence. It also increases the risk of diabetes, which may also affect bladder control. Losing excess weight is a must.

Guidelines
- Three meals daily but drinks only between them. You may prefer to miss out a bedtime drink, but make up in the day.
- NO butter, spread, oil, cream, whole milk or fried food.
- NO made-up meat dishes such as pate, burger, sausage, meat pie.
- NO pizzas or quiches.
- NO chocolate, cake, pastry, avocado, puddings or added sugar.
- NO biscuits except water biscuits and crispbreads.
- Alcohol – one drink daily, preferably dry, if you wish.

It may seem that you are not allowed to eat anything. In fact, you must make sure of adequate protein and carbohydrate – fats will take care of themselves.

NOURISHMENT AND REPAIR

- *Two of these daily*. Meat, chicken, egg, fish (tuna, sardine, pilchard, cod), cheese, cottage cheese or fromage frais, soya, baked beans.
- *Three portions daily*. Bread roll, oatcakes, potatoes, rice, porridge, All-Bran, Weetabix, Shredded Wheat, water biscuits or crispbread.
- *Take freely*. Fruit, salads, vegetables and skimmed milk. Use vinegar, pepper or mustard to bring out the flavour of plain foods.
- *Salads*. Lettuce, endive, celery, tomato, grated carrots or parsnips, Chinese leaves, peppers, cucumber, red cabbage, dandelion leaves.

Suggestions

Breakfasts
1. Three fresh fruits (apple, orange, pear, two plums, banana, six grapes, etc.).
2. Porridge made with water and half a cup of dry oats and moistened with fruit juice or skimmed milk, apple.
3. Baked beans and grilled tomato with one slice of toast (no spread).

Lunches
1. Cottage cheese, salad, crispbread.
2. Ham, tomato and slice of wholemeal bread or a potato.
3. Vegetable soup, brown roll, apple, 2 oz chocolate.

Suppers
1. Casserole of meat, root vegetables, onion, stock cube with no fat, bread roll or boiled potatoes.
2. Chicken, meat, Cheddar cheese or ham, salad.
3. Prawns or chicken, rice and broccoli.

Second course. Pot of yoghurt. Fresh or stewed fruit. Soya dessert. Plain sponge cake, such as is used in trifles, with any of these.

Water or decaffeinated coffee or tea and semi-skimmed milk with each main meal and between meals at midmorning, mid-afternoon and evening (optional).

NOURISHMENT AND REPAIR

Muscle- and tissue-building diet

To repair damage from pregnancy and childbirth, cystitis or other infection in the pelvic area and to build up strength and immunity. The emphasis is on protein and adequate vitamins, but not an excess.

- *On waking.* Tea with milk, sugar if desired, semi-sweet or sweet biscuit.
- *Breakfast.* Juice or an orange, cereal with milk, scrambled or poached egg with ham, bacon, cheese or a kipper, toast with butter or spread and honey, coffee, tea or chocolate with milk and sugar if desired.
- *Midmorning.* Drink as above, shortbread or other sweet biscuit.
- *Lunch.* 3–4 oz (70–100 mg) meat, white fish, hard cheese or ham, or two eggs in a sandwich with salad garnish, tomato or celery, followed by whole milk yoghurt, rice pudding or apple tart, water, tea or coffee.
- *Tea.* Egg, soft cheese or tomato sandwich, plain cake, tea or herb tea.
- *Supper.* Juice or soup, 4 oz (100 mg) meat, fish, cheese, ham or eggs with vegetables or salad, potatoes or half a slice of bread, followed by fruit jelly, baked custard, banana, fruit upside-down cake or cheese and biscuits, small glass of wine if desired, coffee or herb tea.
- *Bedtime.* Small milk drink – plain, chocolate or Horlicks.

The programme is intended for a limited period, and should be tailed off to the general purpose diet if it increases your weight beyond what is your normal, for instance what it was before the pregnancy or illness.

Diet in the menopause

This is the time to review your eating habits, to accommodate changes in your hormones, your metabolism and your lifestyle. You may be at the peak of your professional career or taking on your responsibilities as a grandparent conscientiously.

Points to remember
Now is when you need to get into shape since it is all too easy to bulge into a middle-aged spread and exceedingly difficult to shed unwanted fat after the age of 50. Getting your weight right helps you

NOURISHMENT AND REPAIR

to stay young and you also need to go for the anti-ageing foods – the *antioxidants*. Vitamin E is the principal one and the best sources are:

- spreads with added Vitamin E
- eggs
- wholegrain cereals
- fresh dark green vegetables (spinach, broccoli)
- vitamins C and A

A fundamental effect of the menopause is the drastic reduction in oestrogen. This hormone has a strengthening and protective effect on the pelvic organs, and helps tone up the muscles concerned with continence. Hormone replacement therapy is widely used to compensate for the ovaries' retirement, but it can have side-effects. This is not a problem with the *phyto-oestrogens*, oestrogens from plants. They help harmlessly and naturally when there is a shortage of oestrogen, but are not as powerful as the tablets.

Sources include:

- soya and tofu
- legumes – the pea and bean family, including mung beans and chickpeas
- sunflower seeds, sesame seeds

Pamela
Pamela was a chocoholic. As a teenager she had been curvaceous and cuddly but after she had the twins – both nearly 6 lb – her weight went steadily up. She had always been keen on sport, especially tennis and running, and although she was overweight she remained in control of her bladder until, at the age of 45, she had a nasty attack of cystitis. What should have been temporary incontinence became entrenched.

Pamela's bladder had been irritated by the infection and was under increasing pressure from her extra weight, made worse by her comfort eating of chocolate because of her incontinence. She went to the doctor in the hope of a magic pill, but he was not encouraging. Nothing worked and Pamela could not summon the commitment needed to persevere with pelvic floor exercises. Finally her GP sent her to a urological surgeon. He agreed to operate, but only if Pamela lost at least a stone and a half.

The frequent 'accidents' and the constant changing of pads, with all the awkwardness of disposing of the wet ones, for instance when she was at someone else's house, got her down. When it seemed that her marriage and her family were in jeopardy she finally buckled down to an 800-calorie-a-day diet and succeeded in reaching her target weight. The promised operation, a standard colposuspension, provided the answer to Pamela's incontinence. It took six weeks for her to recover, but now all she has to remind her is a neat bikini-line scar and a restored family life.

Vitamins

It is important to check that your diet contains an adequate supply of these when you are building up your strength, including in the pelvic area, after having a baby or an infection such as cystitis, or suffering menopausal symptoms. However, it can be dangerous to exceed the recommended daily allowance (RDA) printed on food labels. We need the same amount, neither more nor less, throughout our adult life. Although pharmacists' shops are full of bottles of vitamin tablets, they are better absorbed and utilized when they are part of your daily food.

Those relevant to the working of the urinary system are:

Vitamin C
Vitamin C (ascorbic acid) is needed for the manufacture of collagen, elastic supporting tissue that is used in healing skin and other damaged tissues, and in making scar tissue. It is just what is needed for the pelvic floor. It also helps the body to absorb iron. You need 60 mg daily and you find it in fresh fruit, especially blackcurrants and citrus, such as oranges, salads and lightly boiled vegetables such as spinach, broccoli and sprouts.

Smoking, the contraceptive pill, aspirin and steroids inhibit its absorption.

Folate
Folate is particularly important in pregnancy, and liable to run short in older people who live alone on a restricted diet and Asian people who rely on rice. They may develop anaemia, which causes tiredness

and difficulty in concentrating. You get your supply from liver, oranges, lettuce and lightly cooked broccoli, Savoy cabbage and runner beans. Cooking tends to destroy folate, and hormone replacement therapy (HRT), anti-epileptics and too much alcohol interfere with its absorption.

Vitamin B12 (cobalamin)
Vitamin B12 (cobalamin) is unique in that it is not found in any plants. Vegetarians get by on eggs, milk and cheese, but strict vegans survive on germs and moulds contaminating their food. To make matters worse B12 is not absorbed in the presence of colchicines, a treatment for gout, slow-release potassium or a parasite in some Japanese fish eaten raw. The effects of a lack of cobalamin are dire, affecting growth in babies and the blood and nervous system in everyone. Damage to the nerves with loss of control of the bladder can lead to continuous incontinence. All animal products contain B12, but the richest are liver, meat and poultry and normally we never run short. Nuts and legumes make up for some of the shortfall in protein for vegetarians.

Vitamin E
Vitamin E is the leading antioxidant and benefits every cell in the body including the pelvic area. It is most abundant in vegetable oils, especially wheat germ oil, but is also found in nuts and seeds, wholegrain cereals, butter and eggs.

Vitamin D
Vitamin D, the home-produced sunshine vitamin, is made from the oils of the skin by the action of ultraviolet light, most effectively in fair people. It is increasingly important, in conjunction with calcium, from the menopausal years onwards to ward off osteoporosis. Very little of this vitamin is absorbed from food, but a little is present in fish oils and such favourites as sardines, tuna and salmon.

Minerals

Only two minerals are of particular concern in middle age and later – calcium and iron.

Calcium
Calcium is important for healthy bones, but exercise is also essential.

Calcium is lost in the urine as the menopausal dwindling of oestrogen in the blood takes hold. Steroid medicines also lead to a reduction in calcium.

Food sources are dairy products and sardines, and especially fortified white bread, but since 70 per cent of the intake goes out through the bowels, you have to eat and drink plenty of the appropriate foods. An additional problem is the effect of phytates. A fashionable 'healthy' diet with generous quantities of wholegrains, oatmeal and fibre contains phytic acid. This interferes with the absorption of calcium. White bread has no phytates in it, one way in which it wins.

Iron
Iron has a key role in enabling the blood pigment, haemoglobin, to perform its vital task of carrying oxygen to all the tissues of the body. The commonest form of anaemia, very much a woman's disease, is due to iron deficiency. It affects up to 20 per cent of women over 60, but younger women with heavy periods often run into anaemia. Having a baby is a tremendous drain on the iron reserves. Although iron deficiency does not have a direct effect on urinary incontinence its weakening effects on the muscles, especially those of the pelvic organs, makes it more likely to occur and slower to recover from.

Many diets are short on iron – vegetarian, some Asian, those of older people with inefficient dentures, and slimmers. The best absorbed and richest sources are meat and liver. Well behind come oatmeal, All-Bran, legumes, baked beans, watercress, dried figs, sardines and chocolate.

Agnes
Agnes was 77, erect and dignified as befitted a former headmistress, and noticeably thin. This was because of her determination not to ingest more calories than were strictly necessary. She had always prided herself on her self-control, so it was unendurable for her to find that her bladder, nowadays, simply refused to comply with her demands.

Although she tried, Agnes could not get personally involved with the part between her legs, so exercises were not a possibility. She had become incontinent because the neck of her bladder had sagged until it was no longer in the right position for preventing leakage. She had no spare fat packed round the organs in her pelvis to cushion them and keep them in place.

Agnes asked for an appointment with a specialist and he suggested that she might benefit from a bladder neck injection. She agreed at once. It was a simple procedure: the injection of GAX, bovine collagen, a bulking material obtained from cows. The aim was for it to surround and support the bladder neck. Agnes could have had the procedure under a local anaesthetic as a day case, but like most other patients she preferred a general anaesthetic and an overnight stay in hospital. The injection was not a cure, but it made Agnes's incontinence manageable, and if necessary she could have a repeat.

Agnes was one of the few people, apart from anorexics, who would have benefited from eating more and retaining a layer of fat for warmth, cushioning and protection. Diets and food fads can be dangerous if they are extreme in any way. Pamela's downfall was too much chocolate, Agnes suffered from too much austerity, and there are several definitely dangerous diets – mostly aimed at weight reduction.

Diets to avoid

- *Zen macrobiotic diets* come in ten stages – the highest is 100 per cent cereal and very little fluid, which is particularly bad for the urinary system. They can lead to scurvy, kidney damage and even death.
- *Strict vegan diet* causes a lack of Vitamin B12, with damage to the brain and nervous system and anaemia. Development is drastically impaired in babies breast-fed by vegan mothers. Vitamin D is also lacking from a plants-only diet but this vitamin can be manufactured in the skin if it is exposed to ultraviolet light.
- *The Beverly Hills Diet* consists of fruit only for the first ten days, in a special order, and later some salad, bread and meat.
- *Dr Atkins's Diet Revolution* is a popular American reducing diet containing very little carbohydrate. The second edition is safer than the original.
- *'Liquid protein' (Prolinn) plus fasting* caused a number of deaths

from heart failure in the 1970s. Prolonged fasting, even with a protein supplement, can disturb the rhythm of the heartbeat.

Moderation and gradual adjustments when needed are the rule, as with so much in nature.

Further reading

Chiarelli, Pauline, *Women's Waterworks*, Robinson, London, 1995.
Dawson, Chris, and Hugh Whitfield, *ABC of Urology*, BMJ, London, 1997.
Gomez, Joan, *Sixtysomething*, Thorsons, London, 1993.
Mandelstam, Dorothy, *Incontinence*, Heinemann, London, 1977.
McClelland, Joan, *How to Cope Successfully with the Menopause*, Wellhouse, Farnham, 2001.
Smith, Jane, Raj Persaud, Phillip Smith and Ann Winder, *Keeping Control*, Vermilion, London, 2001.
Toozs-Hobson, Philip and Linda Cardozo, *Urinary Incontinence in Women*, BMA, London, 1999.
Toozs-Hobson, Philip and Linda Cardozo, *Understanding Female Urinary Incontinence*, Family Doctor Publications, London, 2002.

Useful addresses

UK

Age Concern England
Astral House
1268 London Road
London SW16 4ER
Tel: 020 8765 7200
www.ageconcern.org.uk
Provides a fact sheet on incontinence.

Association of Chartered Physiotherapists in Women's Health
14 Bedford Row
London WC1R 4ED
Tel: 020 7242 1941
Email: *webmaster@womensphysio.com*
www.womensphysio.com

BMJ Publishing Group
BMA House
Tavistock Square
London WC1H 9JR
Tel: 020 7387 4499

British Red Cross
National Headquarters
9 Grosvenor Crescent
London SW1X 7EJ
Tel: 020 7235 0606
www.redcross.org.uk
Provides incontinence aids and equipment, loans and practical help.

USEFUL ADDRESSES

Continence Foundation
307 Hatton Square
16 Baldwins Gardens
London EC1N 7RJ
Tel: 020 7404 6875
Email: *continence.foundation@dial.pipex.com*
www.continence-foundation.org.uk

Incontinence Information Helpline
Tel: 0845 345 0165
Provides confidential advice from a specialist nurse.

Disabled Living Foundation
380–384 Harrow Road
London W9 2HU
Tel: 020 7289 6111
Text (Minicom): 0870 603 9176

ERIC (Enuresis Resource and Information Centre)
34 Old School House
Britannia Road
Kingswood
Bristol BS15 8DB
Tel: 0117 960 3060
www.enuresis.org.uk

Family Doctor Publications
PO Box 4664
Poole
Dorset BH15 1NN
Tel: 01202 668330

Help the Aged
207–221 Pentonville Road
London N1 9UZ
Tel: 020 7278 1114
www.helptheaged.org.uk
Senior line for advice and information: 0808 800 65 65 (Mon–Fri 9 a.m.–4 p.m.)
Text: 0800 26 92 26
Senior link for immediate telephone response: 01709 389 388

USEFUL ADDRESSES

Incontact
United House
North Road
London N7 9DP
Tel: 0870 770 3246
www.incontact.org.uk
Also *www.pelvicfloor.co.uk*
www.incontact.org.uk
Support network and penpals.

Interstitial Cystitis Support Group
76 High Street
Stony Stratford
Bucks MK11 1AH
Tel: 01908 569169
www.interstitialcystitis.co.uk

PromoCon 2001
Disabled Living
4 St Chad's Street
Cheetham
Manchester M8 8QA
Helpline: 0161 834 2001
www.promocon2001.co.uk

Royal College of Nursing Continence Care Forum
20 Cavendish Square
London W1M 0AB
Tel: 020 7409 3333

The Stroke Association
Stroke House
240 City Road
London EC1V 2PR
Tel: 020 7566 0300
www.stroke.org.uk
Booklet on stroke and incontinence.

USEFUL ADDRESSES

USA

Continence WorldWide
Email: *info@continenceworldwide.com*
www.continenceworldwide.com

National Association for Continence
PO Box 8310
Spartenburg
South Carolina
SC 29305-8310
Tel: 864 579 7900
www.nafc.org

The Simon Foundation for Continence US
PO Box 815
Wilmette
Illinois 60091
Tel: 847 864 3913
www.simonfoundation.org
Contact Cheryl Gartley, President.

Society of Urologic Nurses and Associates
Box 56, Pitman
East Holly Avenue
New Jersey
NJ 080701 0056
www.suna.org

Australia

Continence Foundation of Australia Ltd
GPO Box 9919
Melbourne 3301
North West Hospital
Poplar Road
Parkville 3052
Tel: 61 3 9388 8033
Email: *contfound@mail.gsat.edu.au*
www.contfound.org.au

USEFUL ADDRESSES

National Continence Helpline
Freecall: 1800 33 00 66
(8 a.m.–8 p.m. seven days a week)

New South Wales
Tel: (02) 9840 4165
Helpline: 1800 069 789

CFAACT (Continence Foundation of Australia Advisory Committee)
Tel: (02) 6205 3308

Victoria
Tel: (03) 9388 8022

South Australia
Helpline: (08) 8374 3476

Northern Territory
Tel: (08) 8922 7283
Country Freecall: 1800 814 925 Alice Springs
Tel: (08) 8951 6737

Tasmania/Queensland
Tel: (03) 6222 7303
Freecall: 1800 33 00 66

New Zealand

New Zealand Continence Association Inc.
41 Pembroke Street
Hamilton
Tel: (64) 7 834 3528
Email: *stuart@wave.co.nz*
Contact Jill Brown, Secretary.

Index

accident vii, 33
Ada 88
addiction 116
Agnes 138
alcohol 11, 36, 42
Alice 17
Alzheimer 11, 108
andropause 20
Anne 53
antibiotics 72
anticholinergics 68
antidiuretics 76
antispasmodics 69
anxiety 92
aromatherapy 75
augmentation cystoplasty 79
Avril 107

bedpans 66
bed-wetting 30
biofeedback 86
bladder instability 8
Bobby 37
bubble-bath 2
bullying 4

caffeine 10, 19, 42
calcium 19, 137
cancers 43; bladder 103
Catherine, St vii
Charlie 34
Child Guidance Clinic 37

cigarettes 7, 99 *see also* smoking
citrus 42
Claire 109
climacteric 13
collagen 38
commode 67
cones, vaginal 86
constipation 10, 31, 41, 107
cough 10
cranberry juice 99
CVA 51, 108
cystoscopy 61

densitometry (bone) 29
detrusor 1; myomectomy 79
diabetes 40, 119
dienoestrol 18, 71
diets 130–5; to avoid 139–40
dipstick 102
diuretics 10, 42, 71, 73
dribbling 22, 43
drill, bladder: basic 81; mini 82
dyspareunia 18
dyssynergia 8, 108

Ebers papyrus vii
Edna 115
egg-cell 14
Egypt vii
electromyogram 61
Elizabeth 103

INDEX

enuresis: primary; secondary 30–1
epidural 54, 73, 80
Erica 18
Estelle 36
Esther 76

Fallopian tube 1
fibre 22
fibroid 48, 107
finasteride 22
fistula 9, 47; vesico-vaginal 48; colovesical 48
five-day diary 57
folate 136–7
fomentations 76
frequency 19, 48, 69
Freud viii

Gerald 22
gravity 2
Greta 128
guidelines, dietary 129

haematuria 44, 100
headaches 117
hemiparesis 50
hesitancy 12
hot flushes 17
HRT 47, 71
hyperplasia 21
hysterectomy 48

imaging 60
'in case' syndrome 111
incontinence: stress 6, 52; urge 6, 48; giggle 35; coital 37; overflow 39; faecal 88, Ch 15

insomnia 93, 118
intravenous urogram 60
iron 138

Jeremy 50
Jessica 29
John 58
Joyce 89

Kegel exercises 55, 115
keyhole surgery 77
Kirsty 91
KY jelly 18, 96

laparoscopic surgery 77
limbering 122
Lorna 57
lubrication 16, 18
Lynda 97

Margery 47
menarche 13
menopause 14, 20
menses 14
micturition 2; giggle 35
Middle Ages viii
Molly 89
MRI 61
multiple sclerosis 49, 108

neuromodulation 79
nocturia 40

obstruction 8
oedema 71
oestrogen 14, 38; lack 46
Olivia 19
oesteoporosis 15
overflow 8, 12, 26, 39

INDEX

overweight 116
ovulation 14
ovum 14

pad tests 58
pads 64
Pamela 135
palpitations 17
Patricia 70
Pauline 60
pelvic floor 3; exercises 84–5
perimenopause 13
perineal stimulation 85
Peter and Josephine 125
Phaer, Dr vii
Phyllis 39
phyto-oestrogens 16
pis-en-deux 26
pregnancy x, 11, Ch 9
procidentia 45
progesterone 16, 52
prolapse 4, 45, 90; uterine 45; rectal 45
prostadynia 23
prostatectomy 25
prostate gland 4, 20; cancer 24
prostatism 21
prostatitis 23; acute bacterial 23; non-bacterial 23
PSA 24
pseudo-incontinence 10
puberty x
pubococcygeus 3
pyelonephritis 102

reflex 2, 9
relaxation 20–1
retention 26, 43, 52, 105; acute 26; chronic 26

Rosemary 7
Rule of Five 42

sitz bath 74
sleepers 43
sling, vaginal 77
smoking 42, 74, 103
soiling 31
sphincter 2, 5, 52; artificial 78
Stanley 32
STD 27
stone disease 107
stricture 26, 107
stroke 51
Sue 49
sweats 17

talcum 2
TATT 114
testosterone 16
Tina 57
toileting 33
trimethoprim 73
tumours 43
TUNA 23
TURP 108
TVT 78

ultrasound 61
urgency 7, 22, 48, 61; sensory 8; motor 8
urinals 66
urination 2, 4
urodynamics 58
uroflowmetry 59
uterus 1, 52

vagina 1
vaginal: atrophy 39; occlusion

63; plug 63; sponge 63
vaginitis 40, 48, 71, 98
vasomotor symptoms 16
vitamin D 19
vitamins 136–7

voiding 83; double 83; timed 83; prompted 83

Weight charts 112–13